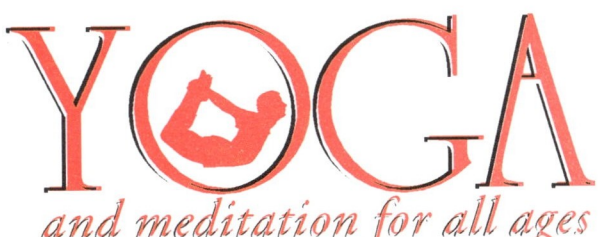

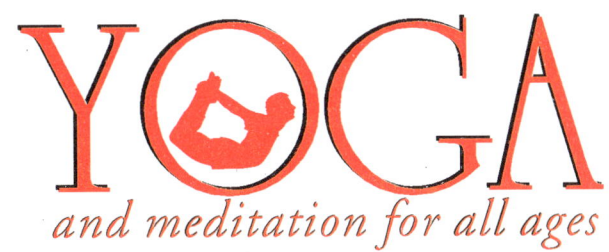

YOGA
and meditation for all ages

BIJOYLAXMI HOTA

RUPA

Published by
Rupa Publications India Pvt. Ltd 2005
7/16, Ansari Road, Daryaganj
New Delhi 110002

Sales centres:

Allahabad Bengaluru Chennai
Hyderabad Jaipur Kathmandu
Kolkata Mumbai

Text Copyright © Bijoylaxmi Hota 2005
Copyright © Rupa Publications India Pvt. Ltd 2005

Photographs: Avinash Pasricha and Sanjay Taneja

Models: Niranjan Koirala, Reela Hota, Dhoop Singh and Reem Ranvita Mohanty
Make-up: Meenakshi Dutt

Thanks to
Swami Swaroopananda Saraswati (Bhubaneswar)

All rights reserved.
No part of this publication may be reproduced, transmitted,
or stored in a retrieval system, in any form or by any means,
electronic, mechanical, photocopying, recording or otherwise,
without the prior permission of the publisher.

ISBN: 978-81-291-0588-2

Fifth impression 2015
10 9 8 7 6 5

The moral right of the author has been asserted.

Designed and illustrated by Ishtihaar, New Delhi

Printed at Yash Printographics, Noida

This book is sold subject to the condition that it shall not, by way
of trade or otherwise, be lent, resold, hired out, or otherwise circulated,
without the publisher's prior consent, in any form of binding or cover
other than that in which it is published.

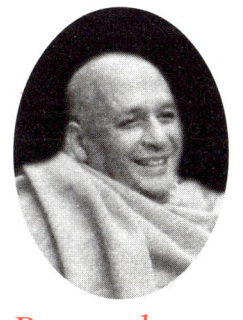

*With the blessings
of my Guru and Guide*

Paramahamsa Swami Satyananda Saraswati

Contents

Why Yoga and When to Start?	8
Yoga at the Age of Five	14
Yoga at the Age of Six	22
Yoga at the Age of Eight	30
Yoga for Teens	36
Yoga for Girls	48
Yoga for Young Adults	52
Pregnancy	62
The Later Years	82
Meditation and its Nuances	96
Yoganidra	108
Nourishment	116
Health Facts	130
References	137
Index	140

CHAPTER 1

why yoga and when to start?

WHY YOGA AND WHEN TO START?

Today yoga is widely practised all over the world. However, not many are aware of its full potential. According to celebrated yogies, yoga can not only prevent and cure all ailments, it can even prevent birth defects.

A human body develops from one cell to trillions of them. During the period in the womb, the inner intelligence, which is the guiding factor for all development, is greatly influenced by the mother's mind. Here, I am reminded of an aunt of mine who was expecting a baby. She had a statue of the one-armed Venus in her living room. Whenever my grandmother visited them, she would object to the statue being there, saying it was not good to see such incomplete figures during pregnancy, and ask them to remove it. My rational uncle would not hear of it, dismissing it as just a superstition. Finally, when my aunt delivered, she gave birth to a healthy boy but with only one arm. Could it be a coincidence? Who can say?

In our body, all functions and developments are controlled by the brain. No cell is completely independent. The brain is not independent either. It is under the control of the hypothalamus which is greatly influenced by the state of one's mind. The hypothalamus can work well when the mind is calm and controlled. But controlling the mind is anything but easy. I remember a gentleman who had come to me with a pain in his shoulder. Tests had revealed no abnormalities. Hence, the doctors dismissed him by saying it was a psychosomatic disorder and he should learn to control the mind and think positive. The gentleman said to me 'I know it is in the mind. I have read all the books on mind control. I have tried all the recommended formulae but of no avail. I cannot get rid of this pain'. After he practised yoga, meditation and *yoganidra* for a few days the pain was much less.

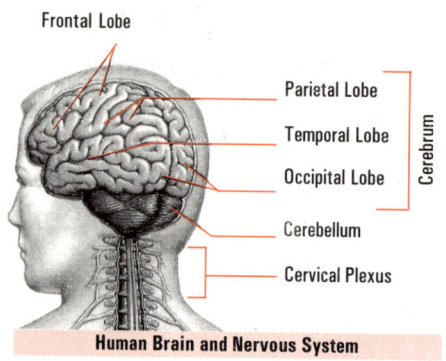
Human Brain and Nervous System

Controlling the mind effectively becomes easier with yoga as *Yogaschitta vritti nirodhah:* 'To block the tendencies of the mind is yoga'. By controlling the mind, yoga controls the brain along with the entire nervous system and thus, all our physical and mental functions.

Yoga can correct many abnormalities, but certain conditions

can be rectified only in childhood and not later, such as:

1. **Scoliosis** is the lateral curvature of the spine. If left untreated it can worsen rapidly and become a permanent problem.

2. **Kyphosis** is the extreme slouch where the muscles of the chest are shortened and their flexibility almost lost.

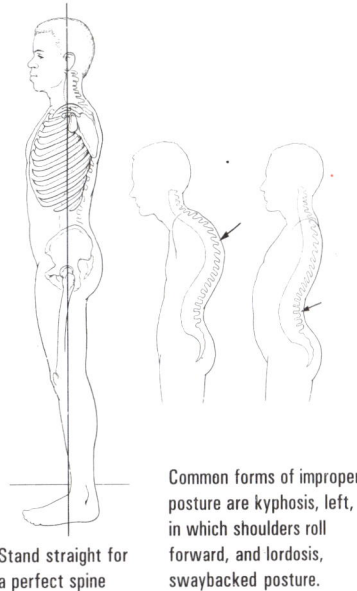

Stand straight for a perfect spine

Common forms of improper posture are kyphosis, left, in which shoulders roll forward, and lordosis, swaybacked posture.

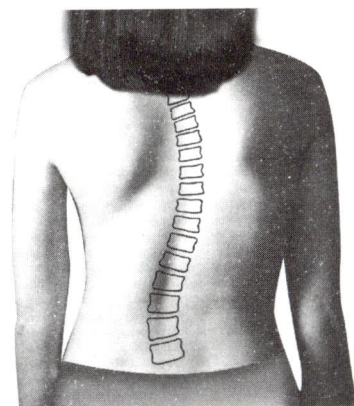

Scoliosis

3. **Cretinism** is where due to insufficient growth hormones a child remains dwarfish.

Often afflictions are labelled as *karmic*, that is, attributed to one's destiny. *Karma* is but action performed, and action is only the transference of one's thoughts, which makes *karma* the ultimate result of one's own thoughts.

According to yoga, various thoughts come to the mind – some significant, some insignificant. The insignificant ones are discarded immediately and are rarely remembered. But certain thoughts make a lasting impression on the mind and keep recurring. These thoughts or *vrittis*, which have a deeper impact on the mind go to the subconscious level and are stored there permanently. They are known as *samskaras* and the sum total of all such *samskaras* is called *karma*.

Karma is not destroyed easily, not even when the physical body perishes. It remains within one's consciousness, and travels to the new body in one's new life and influences one's destiny. To eliminate *karma*, saints and scriptures have recommended certain methods. Some of them are *mouna* (silence), *tapah* (penance), *japa* (*mantra* repetition), prayer, and *dhyana* (meditation). The mind needs to be calm and steady to do any of the above practices successfully and yoga does that effectively.

Thus, yoga not only guards a person's health from birth till death, but if practised from an early age, it ensures proper physical, mental, psychological, emotional and spiritual growth to make one a complete and content human being.

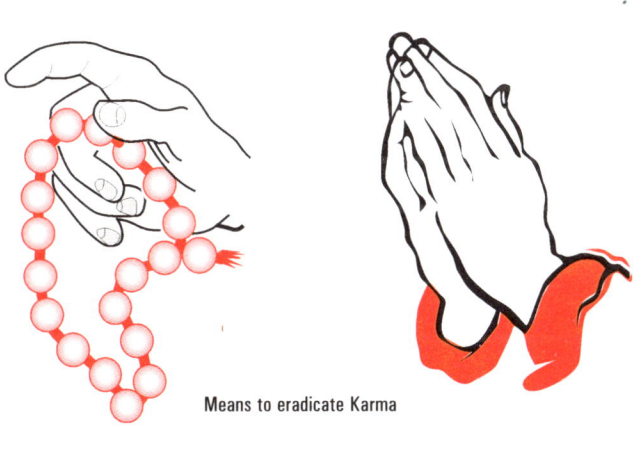

Means to eradicate Karma

CHAPTER 2

yoga at the age of five

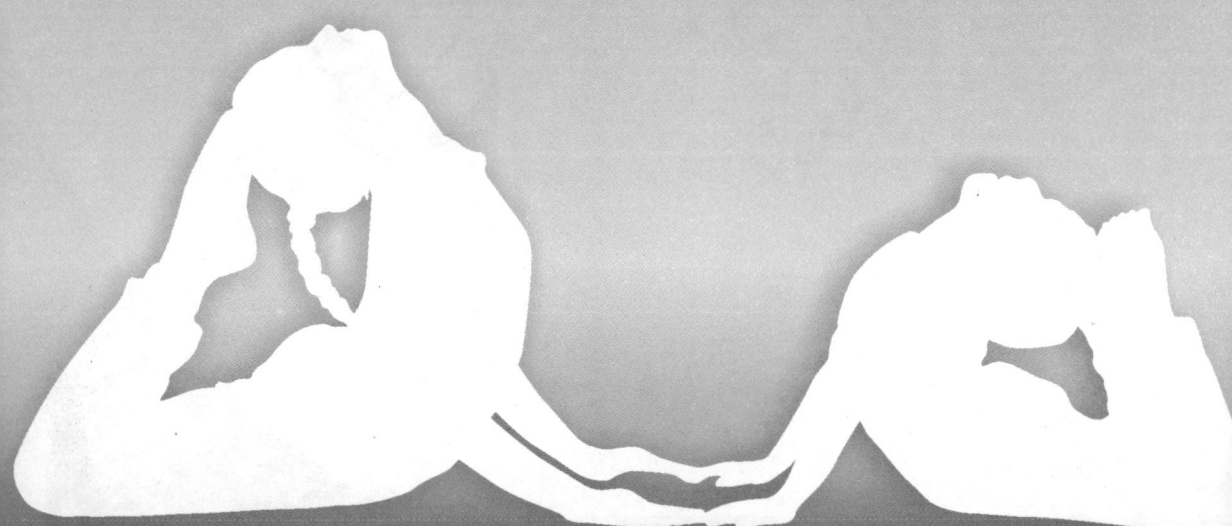

YOGA AT THE AGE OF FIVE

Focus: LUNGS

The human body is composed of trillions of cells, each of which needs oxygen every moment of the day, to live and to carry out its duties. Oxygen is absorbed into the blood and is carried to the cells by the blood, from the inhaled air in the lungs. The more the air in the lungs, the better is the oxygenation of the system. The amount of air one can inhale, depends not only on how one breathes, but also on the size and health of the lungs.

The lungs are made up of tiny air sacs called alvioli. It is here that the actual exchange of gases takes place–the more the number, the more air the lungs can hold. Alvioli growth stops after the age of eight, hence care should be taken for their maximum growth much before that age. The following yogic techniques are extremely effective for this purpose. These techniques also maintain the elasticity of the lungs allowing them to expand fully. With better health of the lungs, the general health of a child improves, preventing various ailments especially of the respiratory system, including asthma.

More Alvioli means better oxygenation

Trachea
Bronchus
Alveoli
Bronchiole

YOGIC PROGRAMME

Simhasana

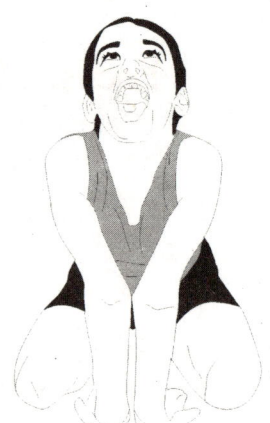

Technique:
- Kneel down.
- Sit on your heels.
- Move the knees apart.
- Place hands on the floor, in between the knees, with the fingers towards you.
- Throw the head back.
- Take a deep breath.
- Open the mouth wide.
- Stick tongue as far out as possible.
- Look up at the point in between the eyebrows.
- Make the sound *aaaaaaaaaaaaa* and expel air from the lungs well.
- Close the mouth and relax your eyes.
- Repeat 10 times.

Makarasana

This asana strengthens not only the lungs but also the back.

Technique:
- Lie down on your stomach.
- Prop yourself up, cupping the chin with the hands.
- Adjust the position of the elbows till you can feel pressure on the mid-back. Remain in this posture for five minutes.

Makarasana can be done as many times and for as long as one wants (in case of an adult, the duration should be increased gradually).

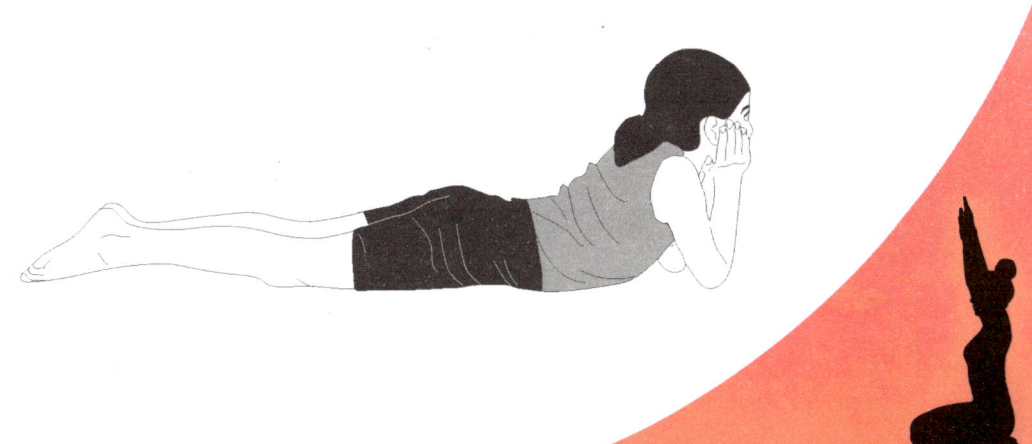

Padmasana (Lotus pose)

Padmasana is known as the destroyer of diseases. It can be done any time and any number of times during the day.

Technique:
- Sit on the floor.
- Put the right foot on the left thigh, and left foot on the right thigh. Place hands on the knees.
- Sit in this position for as long as you can.

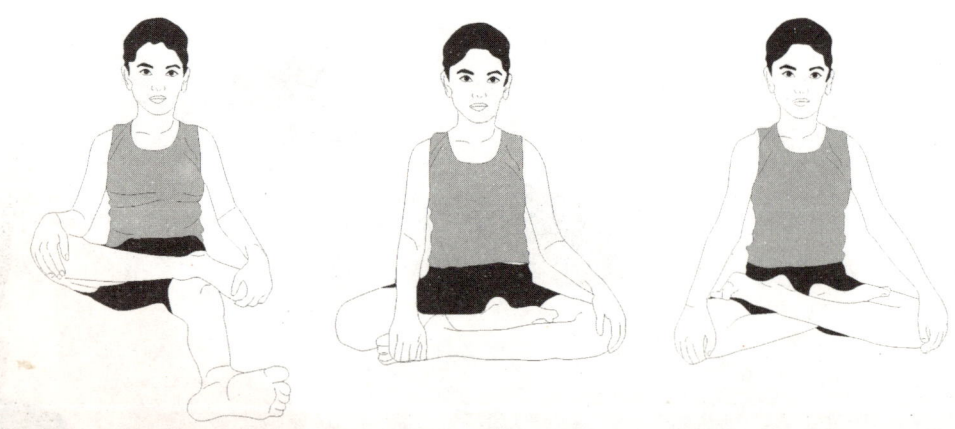

BHRAMARI

Bhramari is a yogic breathing technique or *pranayama*. It expels stale air from the lungs and fills them with fresh oxygenated air. It also soothes and strengthens the nerves.

Technique:
- Sit in *Padmasana* position or just cross the legs.
- Close ears with the index fingers and make a humming sound.
- Repeat 10 times.

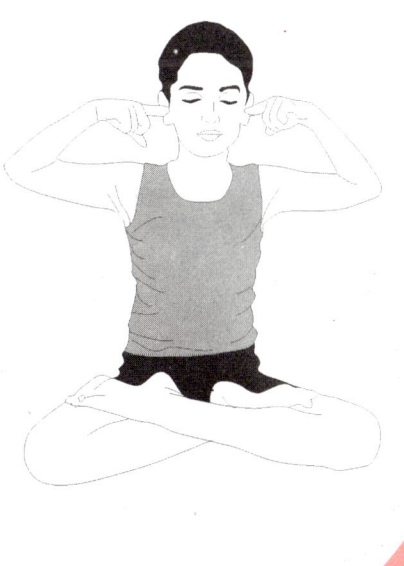

A child of five may not be able to do this perfectly. But he will benefit even if he does it to whatever extent he can.

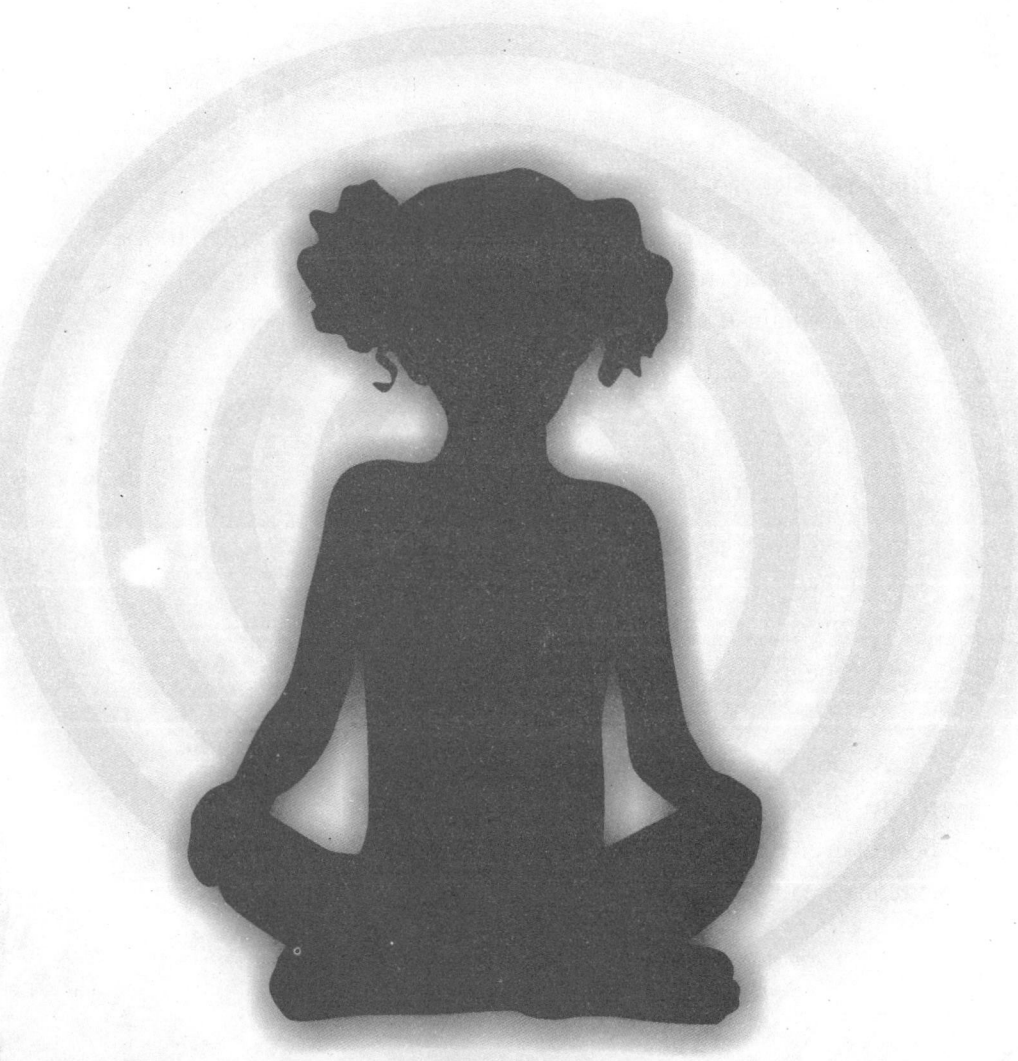

The final routine

Simhasana	page 16	2½	minutes
Makarasana	page 17	5	minutes
Padmasana	page 18	5	minutes
Bhramari	page 19	2½	minutes
Total time		15	minutes

CHAPTER 3

yoga
at the age of six

YOGA AT THE AGE OF SIX

Focus: Memory and Concentration

The formal education of a child starts around the age of six. In today's highly competitive world, even very young children have to work extra hard to keep pace with the demands of the education system, cutting down on their much valuable playtime. Inadequate physical activity can have a detrimental effect on them. A child's motor skills, such as jumping and running, which are refined between the age of six to twelve may also be affected adversely. Mentally too, it may have undesirable effect on the child.

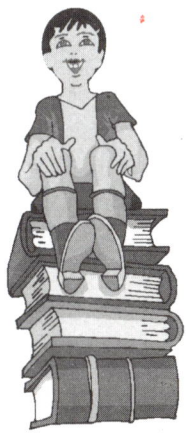

Yoga practised in childhood is a great help to a school-going child, in many ways. First, yoga exercises the body adequately in the shortest possible time. Secondly, it improves the child's memory and concentration manifold enabling him to finish his lessons in much less time than he would otherwise require. This affords him the much needed time for games and sports. And lastly, yoga de-stresses the child's mind and makes him relaxed, cheerful, and balanced – a joy to his parents and everyone around him.

The following asanas tone up the nervous system and improve the memory and concentration.

ANANDA MADIRASANA

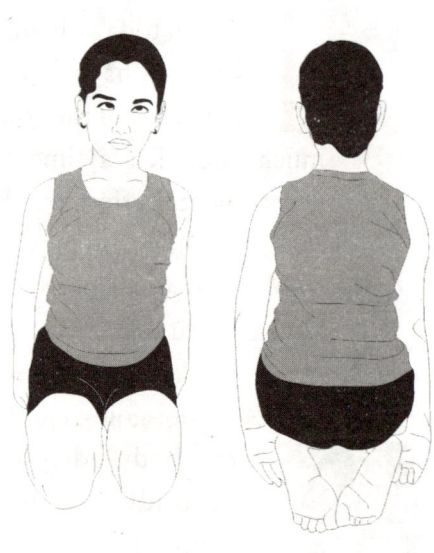

- Kneel down.
- Sit on the heels.
- Hold the ankles.
- Look up and cross the eyes.
- Focus on the point in between the eyebrows (A parent can keep his or her finger a little away from that point and ask the child to focus on the fingertip).
- Take deep breaths. (10 times)
- Close eyes but maintain the posture for half a minute.
- Repeat once more.

Padadhirasana

This asana harmonises the sympathetic and parasympathetic nervous system which leads to activation of higher mental faculties.

- Sitting in the same manner as the previous asana, place the hands excluding the thumbs under opposite armpits.
- Close your eyes.
- Feel breaths in the nostrils, for half to one minute.

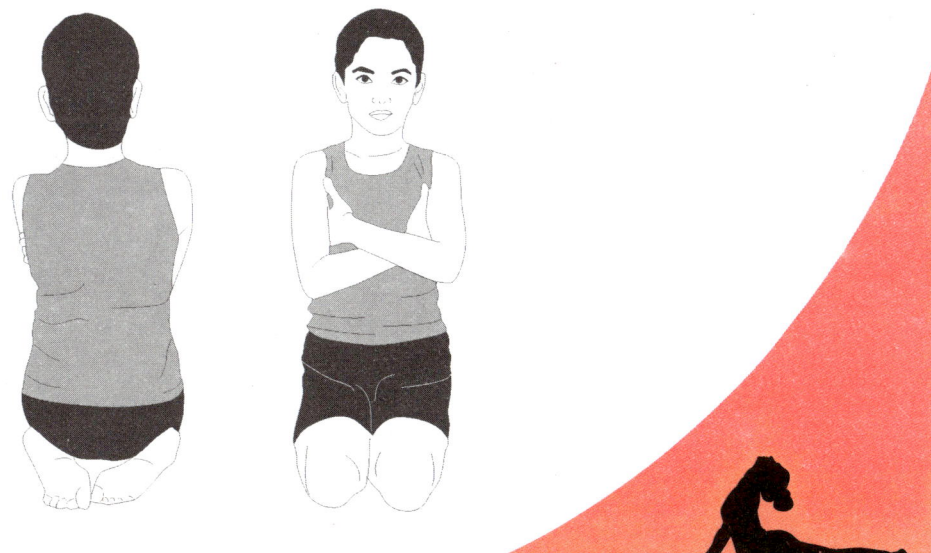

Ekapada Pranamasana

Apart from developing the nervous balance, this asana also strengthens the legs.

- Stand on the left leg.
- Place the right foot inside the left thigh just above the knee.
- Fold hands and keep them near the chest.
- Look straight ahead.
- Maintain the position for half a minute.
- Change the legs and repeat the process on the right leg.

Natavara

- Stand on the left leg.
- Lift the right foot, cross it over to the left side and place it against the left shin two to three inches above the ground. Join the index finger with the thumb of the respective hands.

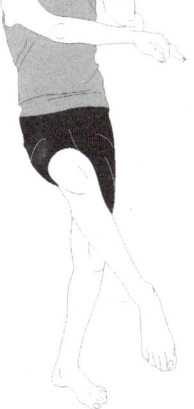

- Hold hands infront of the chest (left hand above the right).
- Standing still, look straight ahead for half a minute.
- Repeat on the other side, keeping the right hand on the above the left.

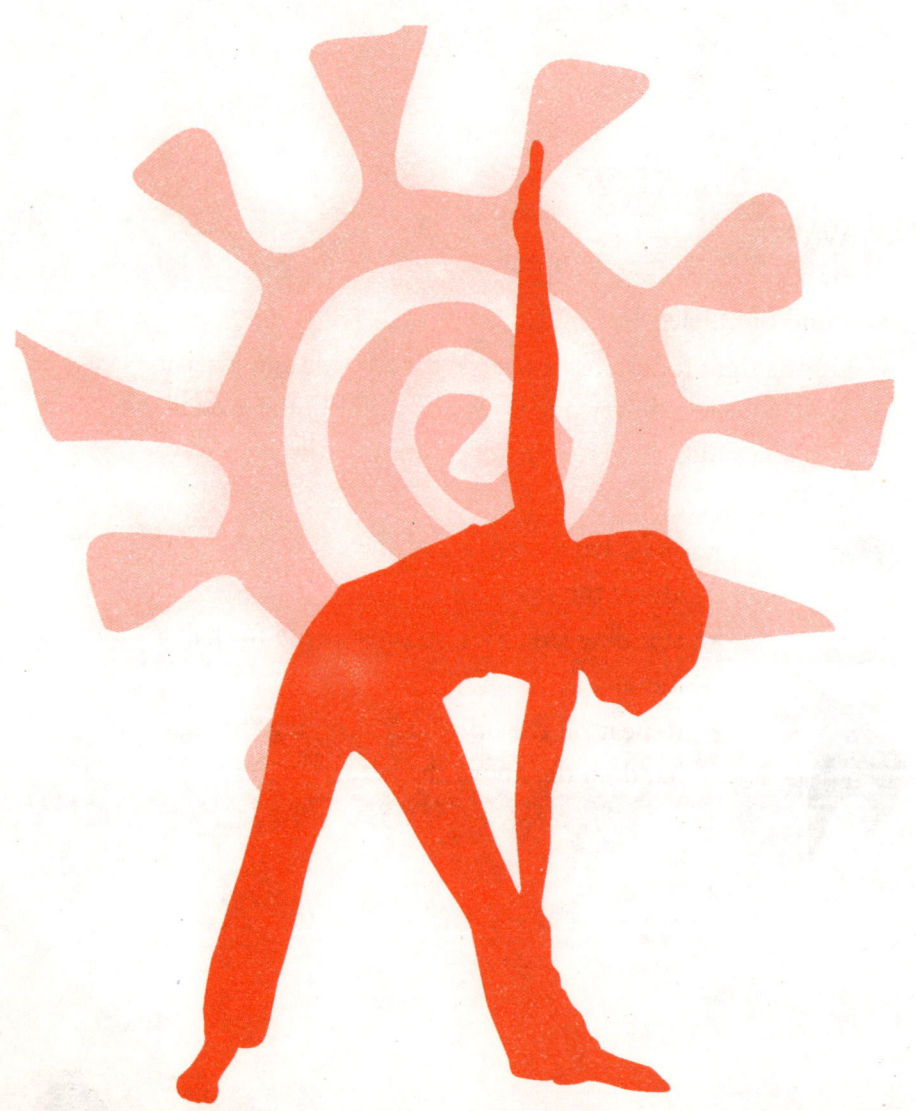

The final routine

Ananda Madirasana	page 24	2	minutes
Padadhirasana	page 25	2	minutes
Ekapada Pranamasana	page 26	1	minute
Natavara	page 27	1	minute
Makarasana	page 17	5	minutes
Padmasana	page 18	2	minutes
Bhramari	page 19	2	minutes
Total time		15	minutes

CHAPTER 4

yoga
at the age of eight

YOGA AT THE AGE OF EIGHT

Focus: Pineal Gland

During childhood, the pineal gland is supposed to keep the pituitary, i.e. the master gland, in check, leading to controlled physical growth of a child. But, when the pineal gland starts degenerating, which normally occurs at the age of eight, its influence over the pituitary gland diminishes. The unchecked pituitary then pours growth hormones into the blood stream, making the child's physical growth rapid. Handling a new body, with its strange urges and desires can prove to be extremely difficult for the child, who is mentally still immature. Certain yogic practices and *mantra* meditation can preserve the pineal health, which then remains active for a longer period delaying puberty. Children can then enjoy a prolonged childhood, and by the time they attain puberty, their minds are mature enough to handle their adult body sensibly.

Perhaps the above mentioned fact was known to Indians in the olden days as *Suryanamaskar* and *Gayatri Mantra* were taught to a child of eight during the thread ceremony.

Surya Namaskar

A group of asanas are put together to form this powerful technique which exercises all the external and internal muscles and glands making them supple, strong and super efficient.

Technique:
Position 1: Stand straight with feet close together and hands folded in front of the chest.
Position 2: Inhaling, raise hands and bend backward.
Position 3: Exhaling, bend forward and place the hands on the floor. You may bend the knees in the beginning.

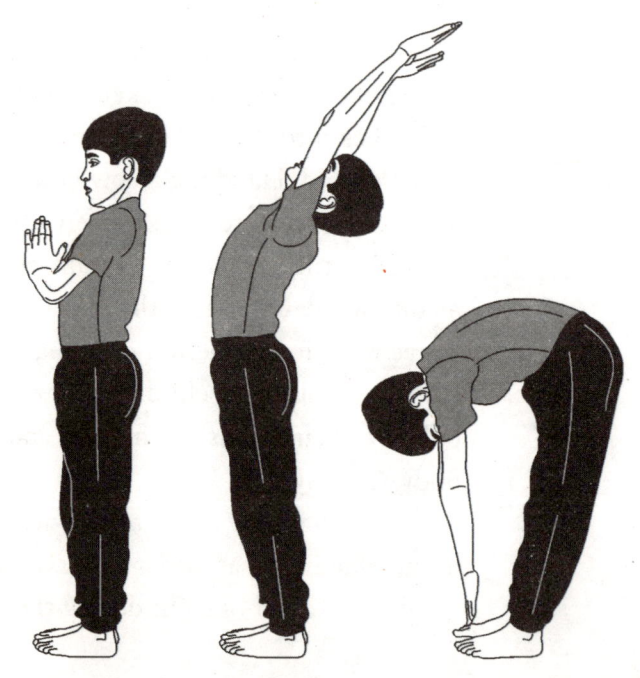

Position 4: Inhaling, stretch the right leg backward, bring the hips down, and look up.

Position 5: Exhaling, take the left foot back to join the right foot.
Lift hips up while keeping the head down.
(The body should form a triangle)

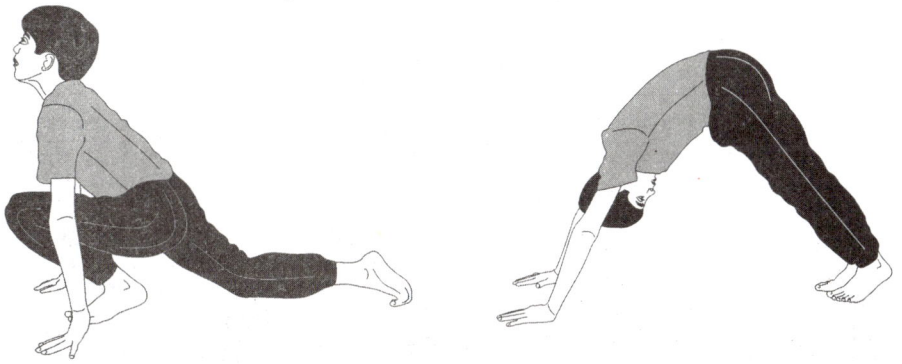

Position 6: Holding the breath, lower the body except the hips to the ground.

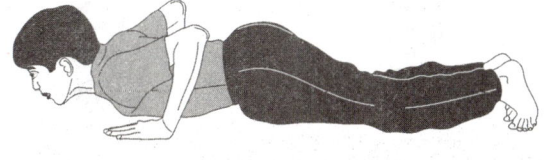

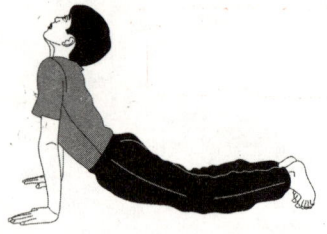 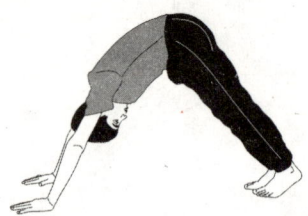

Position 7:   Drop the hips on the floor.
Inhaling, lift head and raise the body from the waist with face turned up.
Position 8:   As position 5
Position 9:   As position 4
Position 10:   As position 3
Position 11:   As position 2
Position 12:   As position 1

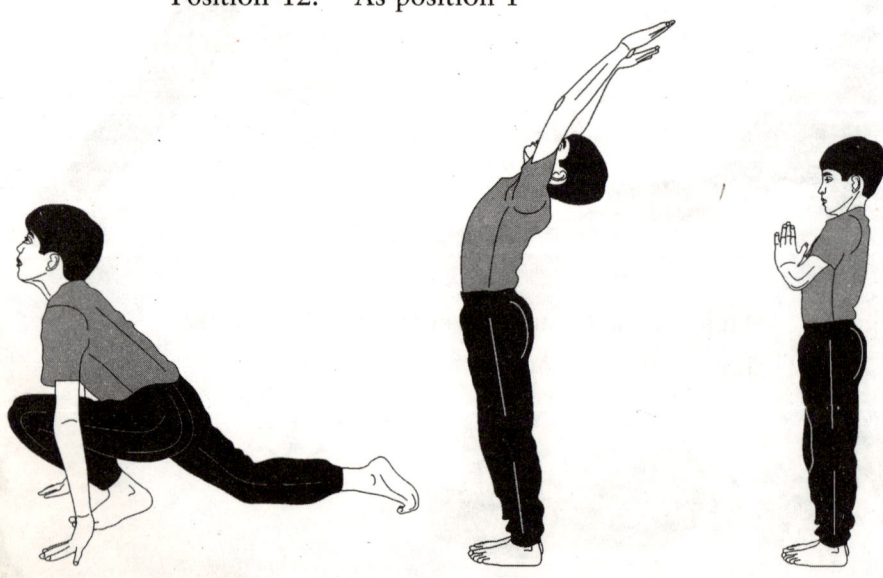

Gayatri Mantra

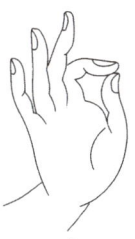

This most revered and popular *mantra* of the *Vedas* is now being recited by children of many nationalities in schools even outside India. Its recitation is said to relax the mind and make it clear. The sound vibration of this *mantra* acts on the body and refines the practitioner's inner nature.

To get the proper benefit of a *mantra*, it is essential to recite it correctly, understanding its meaning is not necessary.

The Mantra
Om bhurbhuvah swah
Tat Savitur Varenyam
Bhargo devasya dheemahi
Dhiyo yo nah prochodayaat

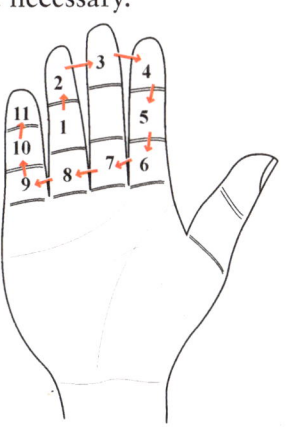

Though reciting the *mantra* even once is believed to be powerful, it should usually be recited a minimum of eleven times.

For counting the *mantra*, touch the indicated points of the palm with the tip of the thumb. This contact can affect the subtle energy of the body in a positive manner.

CHAPTER 5

yoga
for teens

YOGA FOR TEENS

Adolescence – every parent's nightmare! The transition from childhood to adulthood is anything but smooth. Overnight, polite, obedient children turn into monsters. They become defiant, stubborn, and disagree with their parents on almost everything, often loudly and violently. They become painfully self conscious, and imagine that everybody is judging them all the time. Their moods swing wide and fast. They become difficult to handle by family but are easily influenced by friends. With friends, they may indulge in unhealthy activities such as smoking, drinking and experimenting with drugs. At times they may experience intense conflicts with friends which may scar their psyche permanently. Often, teenagers are known to be victims of blinding tempers which sometimes drive them to the world of crime. Adolescents therefore need to be handled with care and sensitivity.

According to yoga, the erratic behaviour and aggression of an adolescent can be due to an unbalanced energy system. There are two kinds of energies in the body – *ida* or mental energy and *pingala* or physical energy. If in a body *ida* is active and *pingala* is subservient, the person becomes quiet and reticent, while a dominant *pingala* gives rise to aggression, violence and destruction. Science holds disturbed glandular function responsible for such undesirable behaviour in adolescent years. For example, an overactive adrenal gland can make a person angry and aggressive, while an underactive thyroid can give rise to depression. A physical problem of the teens, which is also caused due to a disturbed glandular function, is acne. The androgen hormones make the oil glands produce excess oil which blocks the hair follicles. Toxins accumulate there, attracting bacteria leading to infections and inflammation resulting in acne.

The other physical problems which can crop up during the teenage years are:

Vision problems: the rapid physical growth involves every part of the body, including the eyes. Their shape and size may change resulting in impaired vision.

Hearing disorders: listening to loud music – a teenage favourite – can lead to permanent high frequency hearing loss.

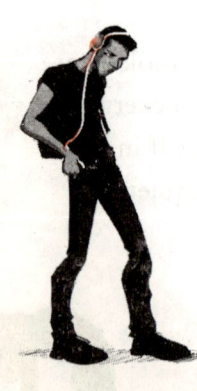

Yogic practices ensure normal glandular functions, soothe the nervous system and strengthen the various body parts including the eyes. Thus, yoga brings about a perfect order in an adolescent's disturbed physio-psychological state.

As teenagers are likely to rebel against taking up yoga, it is advisable to teach them the following practices at the age of ten-eleven, before they are thrown into the turmoil of the teens.

YOGA TO GAIN HEIGHT

The desire to be tall is almost universal. Your chest can be broadened, muscles can be built, weight can be added anytime during your life, but once a person crosses the age of twenty, the height can not be increased by normal means.

Factors determining a person's height are:
(i) Genes
(ii) Diet
(iii) Growth hormones
(iv) Physical activities

Barring the first, all other factors can be manipulated to one's advantage. Proper diet and the following yogic routine are essential for that purpose.

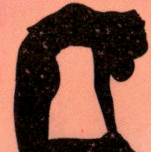

Tadasna

By stretching the spine and the skeletal system this asana encourages the bones to lengthen, adding height.

Technique:
- Stand straight with feet together.
- Interlock fingers and raise arms above the head.
- Inhaling, raise heels and straighten the arms with palms turned out and face turned up.
- Stretch well and hold the posture till you can hold your breath comfortably.
- Exhaling, lower your heels and the hands.
- Rest hands lightly on the head.
- Repeat 10 times.

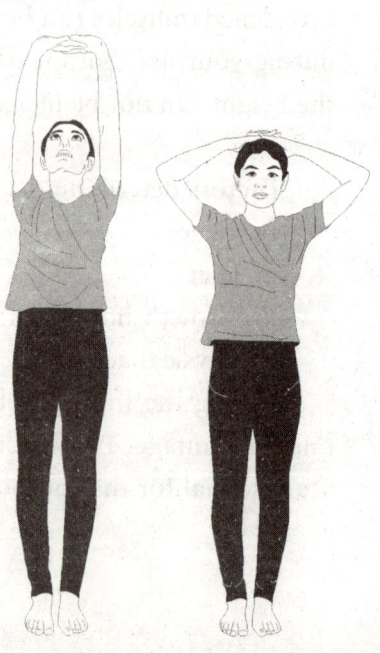

Pada Hastasana

This asana too encourages skeletal growth.

Technique:
- Stand straight.
- Raise hands above the head.
- Exhaling, bend forward and touch the feet.
- Inhaling, straighten the body with hands stretched above you.
- Repeat 10 times.

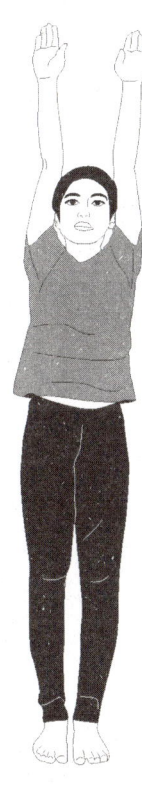
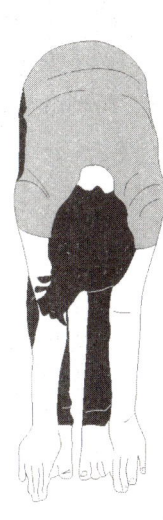
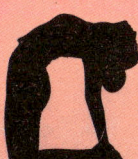

ASANAS FOR STRONGER MUSCLES

DWIKONASANA

This asana helps broaden the shoulders and chest.

Technique :

- Stand straight, holding the hands behind the back.
- Exhaling, bend forward while lifting the hands.
- Inhaling, return to the starting position.
- Repeat 10 times.

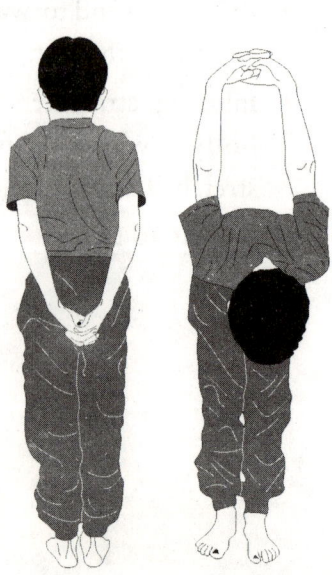

Lolasana

An excellent asana to broaden the chest.

Technique:
- Sit in *Padmasana*
- Place hands on the floor by your sides.
- Inhale and lift your body up from the ground.
- Hold the posture and your breath for some time.
- Exhaling, lower your body to the floor.

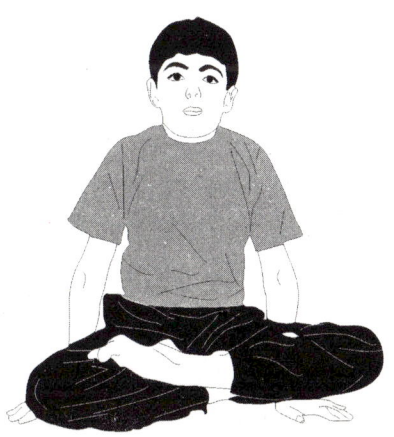

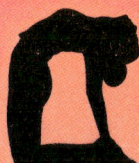

Shashank Bhujangasana

This asana builds up strong muscles in the arms and chest.

Technique:

- Sit in *Vajrasana*.
- Raise hands above the head.
- Exhaling, bend forward and place hands on the floor.
- Inhaling, move your trunk forward, gliding just above the floor till the body is straight.
- Raise head and look up.
- Exhaling, sit back on the heels.
- Inhaling, glide again.
- Repeat 10 times.

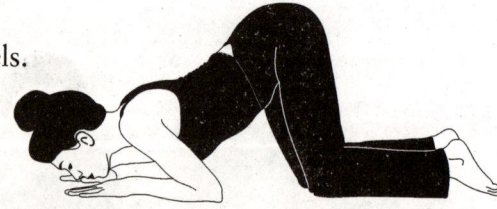

Pranayama should be practised after asanas.

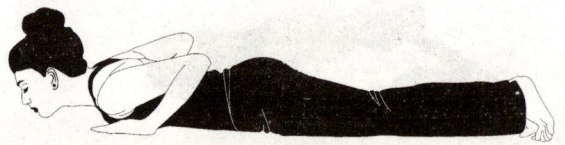

NADISODHANA PRANAYAMA

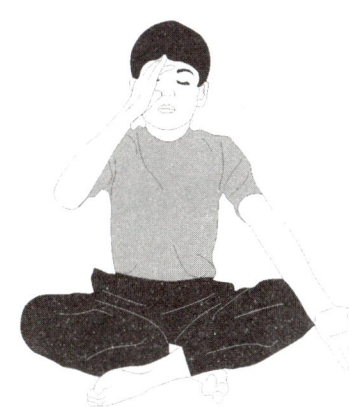

This is a breathing technique which brings about a balance in the sympathetic and parasympathetic nervous systems which in turn ensures smooth physiological functioning.

Technique:
- Sit with your legs crossed.
- Keep the left hand on the left knee with the index finger touching the base of the thumb.
- Place the index and middle fingers of the right hand in between the eyebrows.
- Close the right nostril with the thumb.
- Inhale slowly and deeply from the left.
- Close the left nostril with the ring finger.
- Release the thumb to free the right nostril and breathe out.
- Inhale from the right, close it with the thumb; and removing the ring finger from the left nostril exhale.
- This is one round.
- Repeat each round 10 times.

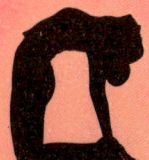

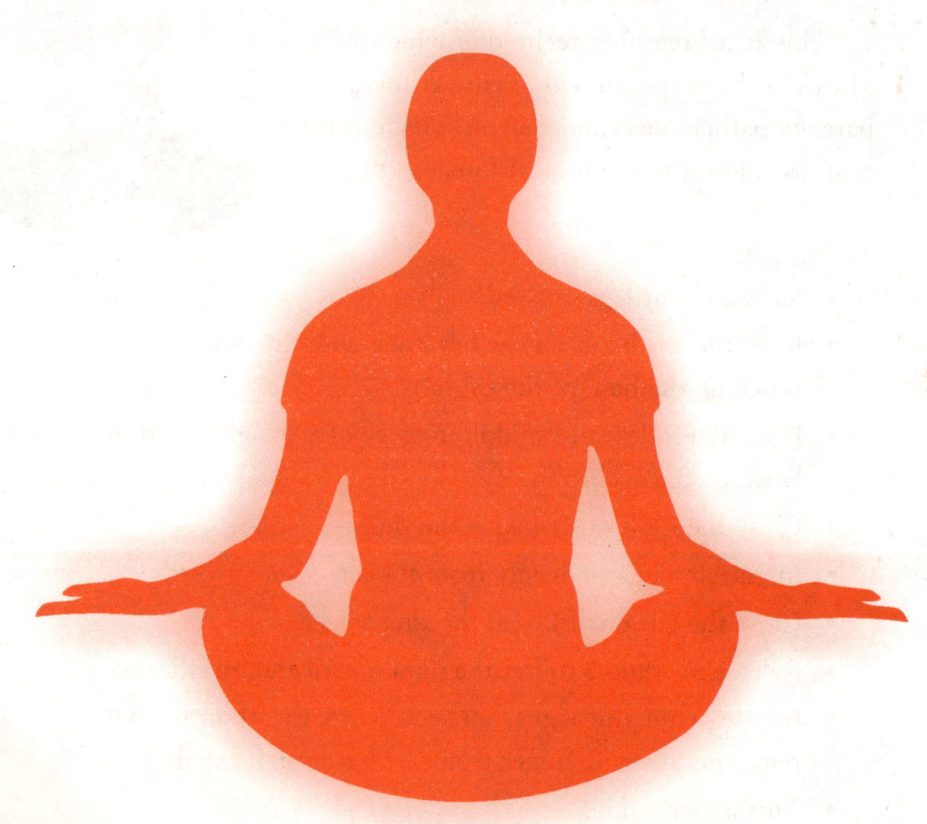

The final routine

Suryanamaskar	page 32	6	minutes
Shavasana	page 113	2	minutes
Tadasana	page 40	2	minutes
Padahastasana	page 41	½	minute
Dwikonasana	page 42	½	minute
Shavasana	page 113	½	minute
Lolasana	page 43	1	minute
Shashanka Bhujangasana	page 44	2	minutes
Shavasana	page 113	½	minute
Nadisodhana Pranayama	page 45	5	minutes
Total time		20	minutes

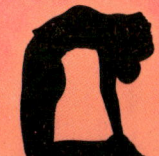

CHAPTER 6

yoga
for girls

YOGA FOR GIRLS

Focus – Uterus

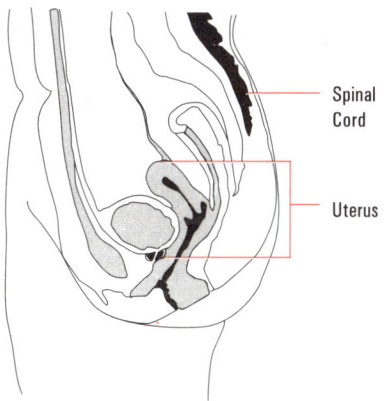

The uterus in a woman's body can cause her much trouble all through her life. She is plagued by the pain and discomfort of monthly periods, pregnancy, childbirth and the problems of menopause. Later in life, uterus may drop from its position and result in a prolapse, causing much discomfort.

The uterus is attached to the lower back with ligaments. During pregnancy, the weight of the growing baby tugs at these ligaments and the muscles of the back, damaging them if they are not very strong. This can result in mild to severe back-ache that can become permanent. Asanas are excellent to strengthen the back muscles, the uterus and the ligaments that carry it.

A girl should be encouraged to practise these asanas from the age of ten or eleven to avoid irreversible damage to the above mentioned body organs.

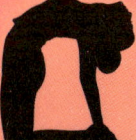

Marjariasana

- Sit in *Vajrasana*
- Extend your arms in front and place hands on the floor.
- Raise the trunk so that you are on all fours. (The arms should be vertical with the hands exactly under your shoulder)
- Inhaling, press the lower back down so the body is concave and tilt the head back to look up.
- Exhaling, lower your head to look down, while arching the back.
- Repeat 10 times.

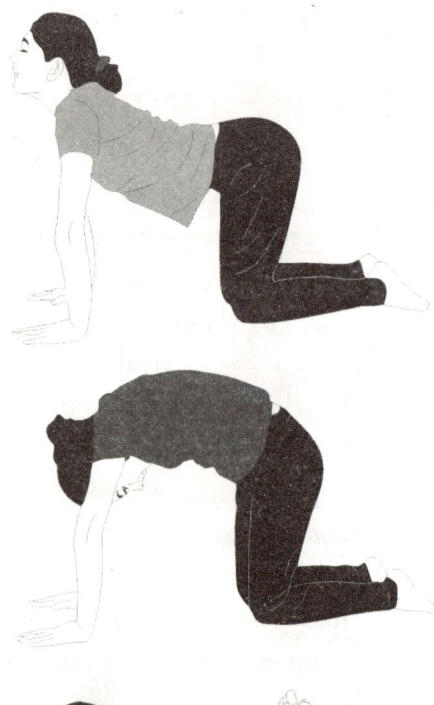

Dhanurasana

- Lie down on your stomach.
- Bend legs and hold the ankles.
- Inhale deeply and lift head and legs.
- Hold the posture for a while.

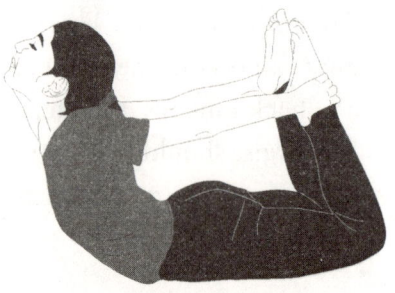

- Exhaling, return to the starting position.
- Repeat 5 times.

The final routine

Surya Namaskar (6 rounds)	page 32	6	minutes
Shavasana	page 113	2	minutes
Marjariasana	page 50	1	minute
Shashanka Bhujangasana	page 44	2	minutes
Rest in Shashankasana	page 59	1	minute
Shavasana	page 113	½	minute
Dhanurasana	page 50	1	minute
Shavasana	page 113	½	minute
Nadisodhana Pranayama	page 45	5	minutes
Total time		19	minutes

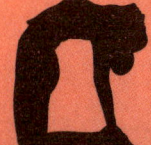

CHAPTER 7

yoga
for young adults

YOGA FOR YOUNG ADULTS

Focus: All Round Health

The confusions, indecisions and mood swings of the adolescent years are left behind when a youth enters a new phase of life with marriage or a job. This phase is marked by a sense of security, stability, financial freedom and a vibrant social life.

Drinking, smoking and late nights become a part of one's daily routine. Such a lifestyle, when overdone, can have undesirable effects on the internal organs, namely the heart, lungs, liver and kidneys. And stress only adds to these problems. The robust young adult may not show the signs immediately but internally the strain continues to weaken the system. Later in life high blood pressure, heart attack, diabetes and liver cirrhosis may surface. What you do in your twenties and thirties definitely does come back to you in your forties and fifties.

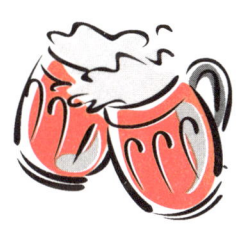

Practising yoga at this stage has many benefits. First, it strengthens the liver and diminishes the harmful effect of alcohol on it. Secondly a youth can practise almost any asana, which may not be possible for an older person. And so, if there is any damage to any organ in a young person, it can be quickly and completely healed and much faster than an elderly person. Thirdly, owing to the good health of youth, the young adult need not practise too many asanas. A few all round asanas that maintain the health of all body organs are sufficient. Later in life when too many body organs have become weak, one needs to practise many more asanas to strengthen each of them. The following are the asanas for a youth with no ailments.

SARVANGASANA (SHOULDER STAND)

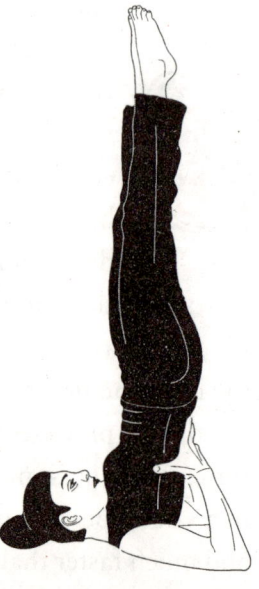

This asana stimulates the thyroid gland and maintains its health, ensuring perfect metabolism. The thymus gland too is stimulated, boosting up the immune system. *Sarvangasana* prevents many male and female reproductive system ailments, such as impotence, hydrocele, prolapse and menstrual and menopausal disorders. Also the extra blood flow to the brain during this asana enhances mental functions.

Technique:

- Lie down on your back. Holding the trunk with both hands, lift the body up to a vertical position.
- The head and shoulders remain firm on the ground with the chin pressed against the chest.
- Hold the posture for a few seconds, and breathe normally. (Never turn your head in the final position.)
- After the desired duration, bend legs and lower the hips, and lie down in *Shavasana*.
- Try not to lift the head while you return to the floor.
- This asana is practised only once.
- The duration should be increased gradually from a few seconds to three to five minutes in the final position.

Sarvangasana should be preceded by *Dhanurasana* and followed by *Matsyasana*.

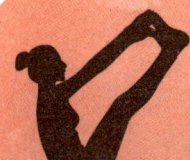

Matsyasana

This asana improves the health of all the abdominal organs and the lungs. The spine too is strengthened.

Technique:
- Sit in *Padmasana*.
- Arching the back and supporting yourself with the arms, bend backward and place the top of the head on a folded blanket.
- Hold the toes and breathe deeply.
- After a few seconds return the same way to the upright position.

Gradually increase the duration in the final position till you can hold it for half the duration of *Sarvangasana*. Those who cannot do *Padmasana*, can practise simple *Matsyasana*.

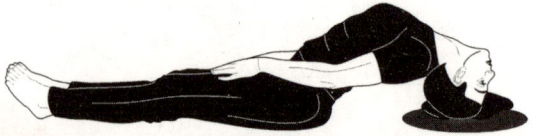
Simple Matsyasana

Paschimottanasana

This is the best asana for the liver.

Technique:
- Sit with your legs stretched in front.
- Inhaling, raise the arms.
- Exhaling, bring them down and bending forward hold your toes – if that is not possible, hold your ankles or calves.
- Hold the posture and breathe normally.
- Start with a few seconds and go up to a minute in the final position.

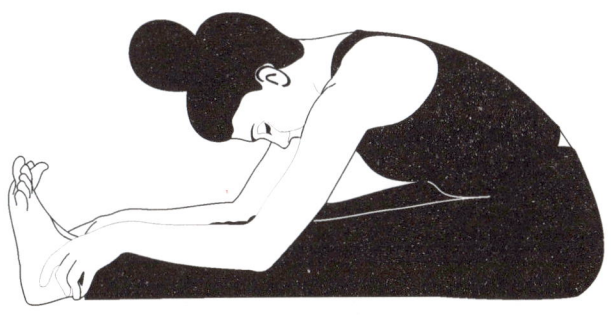
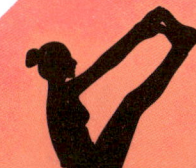

Ardhamatsyendrasana

An excellent asana for the kidneys and pancreas.

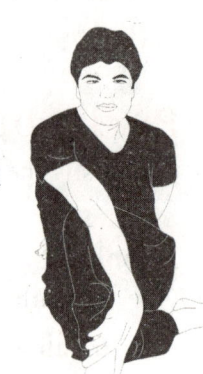

Technique:
- Sit with your legs stretched in front.
- Bend the right leg and place the right foot near the left hip.
- Bend the left leg but keep it upright in front.
- Keeping the right arm outside the left knee hold the left ankle.
- Take the left arm back and encircle the waist, palm turned out.
- Take a deep breath.
- Exhaling, turn the torso to the left, and look over the left shoulder.
- Hold the posture and breathe normally five times.
- Inhaling, return to the starting position.

- Change position and practise on the other side.

Gradually increase the number of breaths to 20 in the final position.

SHASHANKASANA

This asana controls the adrenal gland and calms an angry mind.

Technique:
- Sit in *Vajrasana*.
- Raise arms above you.
- Exhaling, bend forward and place the forehead and forearms on the floor.
- Inhaling, return to the starting position.
- Repeat seven or ten times.

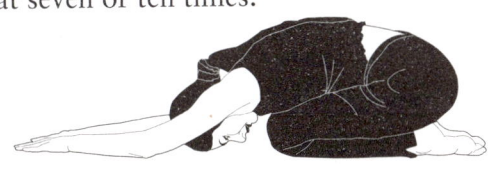
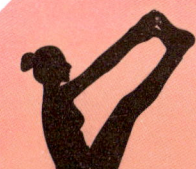

The final routine

Suryanamaskar 6 rounds	page 32	6	minutes
Shavasana	page 113	3	minutes
Dhanurasana	page 50	1	minute
Sarvangasana	page 54	5	minutes
Shavasana	page 113	½	minute
Matsyasana	page 56	2 ½	minutes
Shavasana	page 113	½	minute
Paschimottanasana	page 57	1	minute
Ardhamatsyendrasana	page 58	2	minute
Shashankasana	page 59	1	minute
Shavasana	page 113	½	minute
Nadishodhana Pranayama	page 45	5	minute
Total time		28	minutes

A woman can include *Marjariasana* before *Dhanurasana*.

Additional practices

Gurushankhprakshalana should be performed once a year to wash out the intestine and the harmful substances lodged in the body tissues. This practice also rests and rejuvenates all the over-strained organs.

Laghoo Shankhprakshyalan should be practised at least once a fortnight if not every week, to maintain cleanliness.

(Details of the above mentioned practices are given in the book *Yoga for Busy People* by the author.)

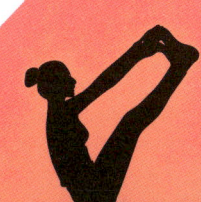

CHAPTER 8

pregnancy

PREGNANCY

Pregnancy is a great responsibility. Not many may be aware of the fact that the physical, mental and psychological health of a child, to a great extent rests with the pregnant mother. It is her health that determines the child's health and it is her thoughts and emotions that shape the mind and psyche of her child. I have experienced it personally.

In my small peaceful hometown, communal feelings are totally absent. All religions are treated equally and there have never been any riots or communal violence. But strangely, I developed an intense fear for a particular religious community which I never discussed with anybody.

I grew up with that fear, married and had children. Once, much later, I was travelling down south with my parents, and we booked into a hotel at night. In the morning, I threw open the windows of my room and lo and behold! Right in front, barely ten meters away from me, was a huge place of worship of that religion. I literally froze; blood drained from my face. My mother, who saw this change, was most concerned and perplexed. When she asked me the reason, for the first time in my life, I told

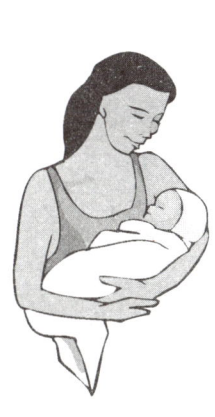

her about my fear. After thinking over it for some time, she came up with the following explanation.

Long ago, when she was pregnant with me, riots broke out in Calcutta. My father, who was studying there, went missing. Fearing the worst, my young mother was distraught. She neither slept nor ate well, and started suffering from terrible nightmares, which continued throughout her pregnancy, even though my father returned home safely after a few days. Her fear was passed on to me since I was a part of her then.

Recognising the cause is the beginning of a cure. Once I realised the reason for my unfounded fear, I felt much relieved. I started practising intense meditation to remove the deep-rooted impression and succeeded. I was thus able to free myself from such a terrible emotion. But, millions throughout the world live nurturing various negative emotions all their lives, and spreading misery and unhappiness all around, perhaps just because their mothers carried negative emotions during their pregnancies.

Perhaps, the influence of a woman's mind on her progeny was well known to the ancient Indians, which is why many ceremonies were performed to make her feel happy. They started even before her pregnancy, with *garbha dhaarana,* where, amidst chants and music, the man approached his wife, bejewelled and sitting under a bedecked canopy, to ask her consent to become the mother of his children. How important and nice the woman must have felt! Another ceremony was *Simontanayana*. It was performed in the fourth or fifth month of pregnancy, where the husband himself adorned the wife elaborately. The scriptures also instructed the husband to take care of his pregnant wife in various ways and to keep her cheerful by fulfilling all her wishes.

Though the husband's cooperation is necessary to keep his pregnant wife happy, she should also practise meditation and release all negative emotions. At the same time, *asanas* and *pranayama* should be practised to remove tension from the body and infuse it with abundant oxygen and *prana* for the better health of the mother and her baby.

FIRST TRIMESTER (three months)

In the first trimester, one should practise all the *asanas* and *pranayama* meant for the young adult. It is a misconception that yoga practice during this period can lead to abortion, as can be seen from the following example.

Long ago, Rinku, a friend of mine, wanted to learn yoga from me. I happened to be very busy at the time and couldn't possibly take out the time to teach her. She did not want to wait for long as her husband, a Foreign Service Officer, was due for a transfer abroad. On my suggestion she went to the ashram in my hometown where she was made to practise all sorts of *asanas* – some rather dynamic ones. Though she had just conceived, that too after a number of miscarriages, she had absolutely no problem. After her full term, she delivered a bonny baby, who is now a robust and brilliant young man.

SECOND TRIMESTER (fourth to sixth month)

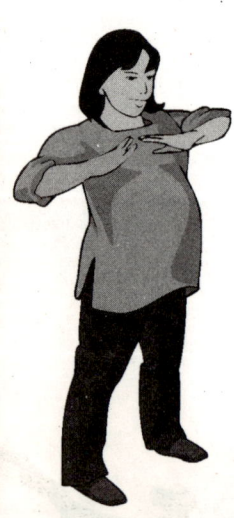

Hindu scriptures say that the soul or consciousness enters the foetus' body in the fourth month. From this time onwards, the mother should guard her thoughts most carefully. She should practise *Yoganidra* and meditation to remain calm and peaceful.

Constipation is a common problem at this time which can be countered with *laghoo shankh prakshalana* while *Kunjal* takes care of morning sickness

(For these two practices – see *Yoga for Busy People* by the author)

Asanas that require lying down on the stomach should be avoided from now on. The following *asanas* are safe to practise during the second trimester.

TITLI

Technique:
- Sit down - bending the legs, join the soles.
- Keep your feet as close to the body as possible.
- Hold feet with both hands.
- Pull up your body.
- Move legs up and down rapidly.
- Practise it for a minute or two.

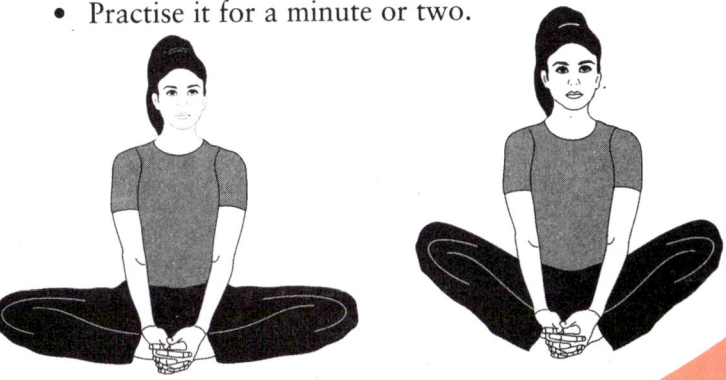

Chakki Chalana

Technique:
- Sit with legs extended in front.
- Interlock the fingers.
- Exhaling, bend forward while moving the arms in a semicircular movement.
- Inhaling, bend backward and bring the hands close to your body bending them.
- Repeat ten times clockwise and ten times anti-clockwise.

(The action imitates the grinding of a hand-mill)

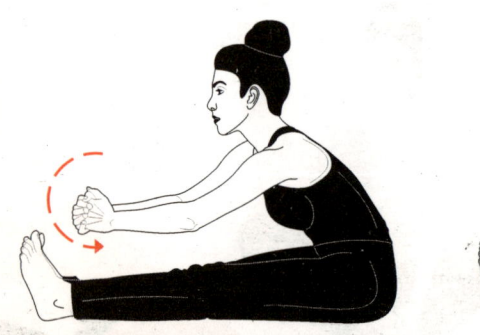
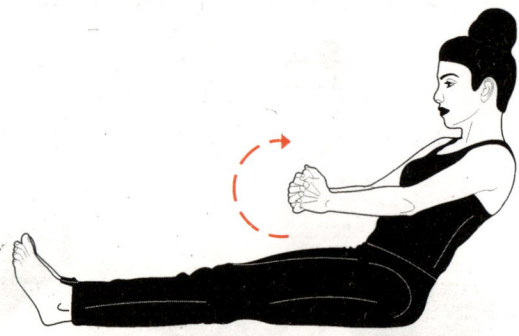

Nauka Sanchalan

Technique:
  Same as the previous asana but instead of moving the arms sideways, they move up and down like the rowing of a boat.

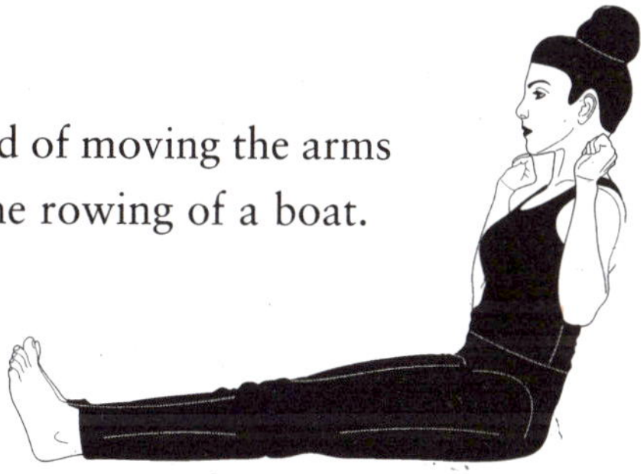

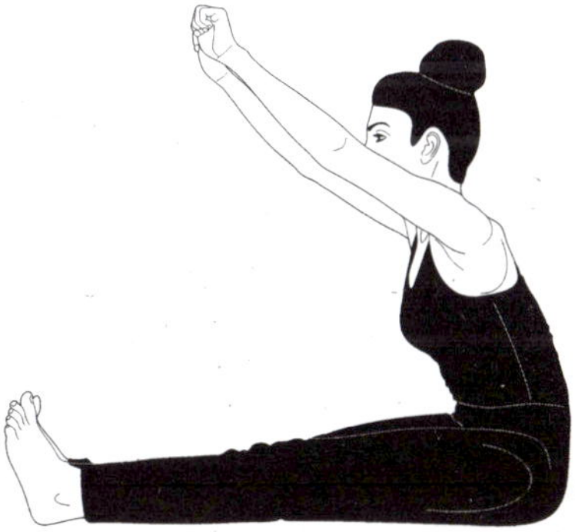

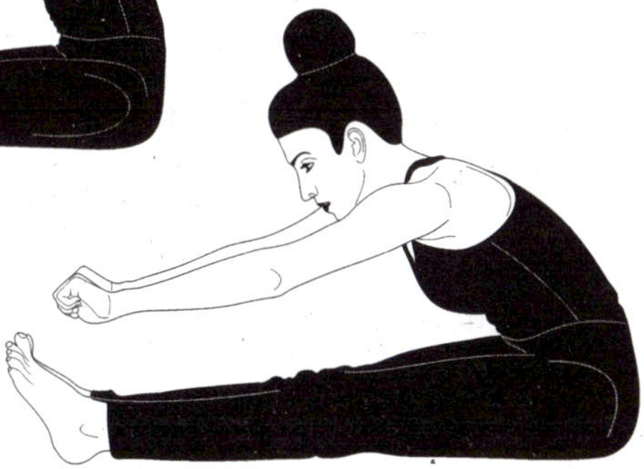

Bhadrasana

Technique:
- Sit in *Vajrasana*
- Retaining the position of the toes, move legs as far apart as possible.
- Breathe slowly and deeply for a minute or two.

Utthanasana

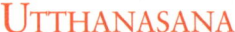

Technique:
- Stand with feet apart.
- Hold hands in front, interlocking the fingers.
- Exhaling partially, lower the body a little by bending the legs.
- Inhaling, return to the upright position.
- Exhaling, lower body half way down.

- Inhaling, return.
- Exhaling, lower the body three quarters down. Inhaling, stand up.
- Exhaling, go all the way down.
- Inhaling, stand up
- Repeat five rounds.

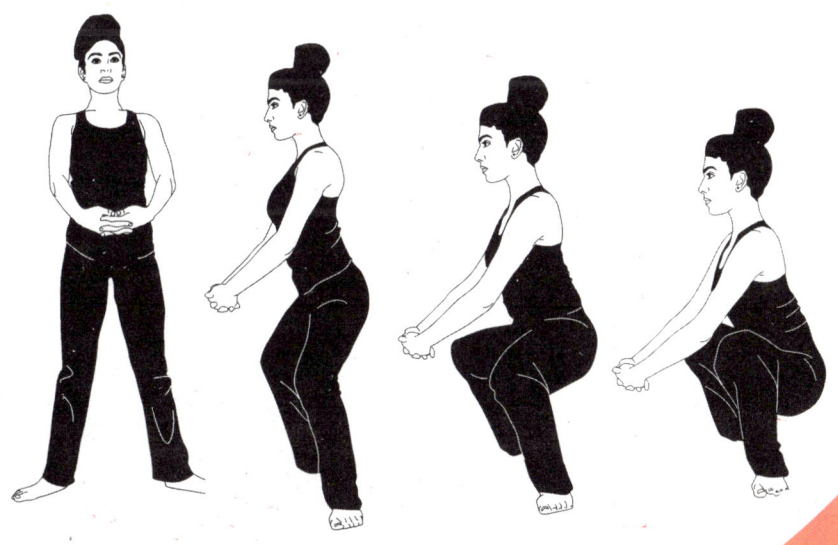

Kandharasana

Technique:
- Lie down on your back.
- Bend legs and bring feet close to the trunk. Place them beside the hips.
- Hold ankles.
- Inhaling, lift the pelvis up.
- Hold the posture for a few seconds.
- Exhaling, return to the starting position.
- Repeat five times.

Gradually increase the duration and hold the final posture for as long as you can hold your breath.

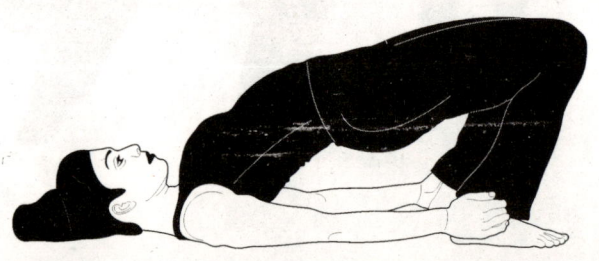

Namaskara

Technique:
- Squat on the floor.
- Join hands and keep the elbows against the thighs.
- Inhaling, push the thighs outwards with the elbows while bending the head backwards to look up.
- Exhaling, push the arms inward with the thighs while bending the head down.
- Repeat 10 times.

After the 4th or 5th month, lying on the back should be avoided as that might restrict blood flow to the fetus. Try to sleep on the side or better still use *Matsyakridasana*. It relieves the pressure from the sciatic nerves and the lower back. Practise it several times during the day.

Matsyakridasana

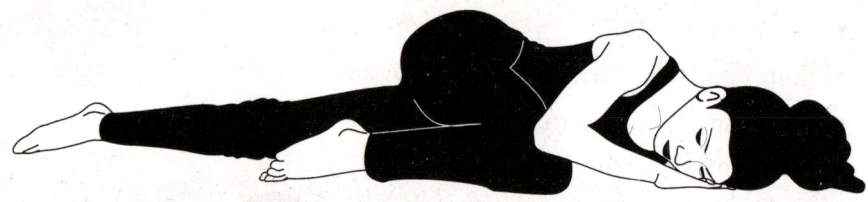

Technique:
- Lie down on your left side.
- Bend the right leg and place the knee on the ground near your chest as high up as possible.
- Interlock the fingers.
- Place the right elbow on the right knee, and the left elbow under the head.

  (The position of the arms may be adjusted to a comfortable position).

The final routine: (second trimester)

Titli	page 67
Chakki Chalana	page 68
Nauka Sanchalana	page 69
Shavasana	page 113
Bhadrasana	page 70
Marjariasana	page 50
Namaskara	page 73
Shavasana	page 113
Utthanasana	page 70
Shavasana	page 113
Kandhrasana	page 72
Shavasana	page 113
Nadisodhana Pranayama	page 45

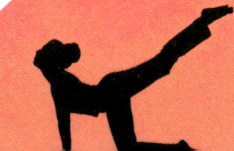

THIRD TRIMESTER (LAST THREE MONTHS)

After the sixth month of pregnancy all the major asanas should be discontinued. *Pawan Muktasana* series (see *Yoga for Busy People*) and *Pranayama* should be practised.

Labour and delivery – A pregnant woman is bound to feel scared at the very thought of labour pains. The fear makes the body tense, including the uterus. This results in more pain, which in turn makes the woman more tense. Soon a vicious cycle is formed and the pain becomes increasingly intense which lasts much longer than normal. For a painless delivery, relaxing the uterus is the first step which is achieved through *Yoganidra*.

To conserve the energy in the body which can get thoroughly depleted with long hours of labour, abdominal breathing (see *Yoga for Busy People* by the author) is excellent. Beside being a relaxation technique it brings more *prana* and oxygen into the system. Another breathing technique called *bhastrika* also de-stresses and energises the body. I noticed my pet cat breathed in a similar fashion when she delivered her babies. In fact, many yogic practices were formulated by observing nature, especially the animal world.

The following method is a combination of *Yoganidra*, *bhastrika* and abdominal breathing which ensures a smooth and easy delivery.

Technique:
- Sit in a meditative position such as *Sukhasana* (cross legged) or *Vajrasana* at the first sign of labour pain.
- Take a deep breath.
- As you exhale chant a long om as *Ooooo – uuu-mmm*....
- Repeat 54 times.

Then lie down in a comfortable position and practise *Yoganidra*. After that you can continue with your normal activities but keep repeating your personal *mantra* in your mind. If you do not have a *mantra* of your own, repeat *Om* mentally. Continue repeating the *mantra* for ten minutes every hour till the pain starts coming frequently. Then you should lie down and follow the following steps:

(i) When the contraction starts, practise abdominal breathing.

(ii) When the pain peaks, practise mild *bhastrika* (panting slightly through the mouth).

(iii) As the pain recedes sigh deeply from the mouth.

(iv) During the relaxed period practise only the first part of *Yoganidra* (moving the mind over the body parts) rapidly.

Continue rotating your consciousness over the body parts till the next contraction and start again from step 1.

Towards the end, when one contraction merges with the next, only continuous panting can be done, till you are asked to push, which you can do effectively with a higher energy level. And the relaxed uterus with strong muscles will push the baby out with much ease. Many women have been amazed at the efficacy of this system. So will you be!

AFTER DELIVERY

Many changes - hormonal and otherwise - take place in the body of the new mother, which may lead to some unpleasant symptoms such as constipation, involuntary urination and pain in the abdomen. Mentally too, a woman might be affected adversely which can make her depressed and/or irritable.

I am reminded of an Austrian lady who had come to India to find a cure for a peculiar problem of hers. She felt that, her *chakras* or energy centres were all open, through which disturbing energies from people around her were entering her body. She was always tense, did not sleep well and generally avoided people. She was so miserable that she wanted to commit suicide, but was afraid to do so as she thought that her *karma* would follow her to her next life to make her miserable then too. She wanted to finish with her *karma* in this life. In India, she consulted a regression therapist who, through hypnosis, took her to her infancy. The lady saw herself as a baby crying in her crib with her mother shouting 'I wish the baby was dead!' Perhaps the mother did not mean what she said. Perhaps it was her low energy and lack of rest that made her speak such harsh words. But it ruined the future life of her daughter.

With yoga, the wear and tear of the body is repaired quickly restoring the depleted energy, while meditation and *yoganidra* help to keep the mind calm, relaxed and reasonable. A woman who turns to yoga soon after childbirth is thus well equipped, physically and mentally, to care for her baby with more patience and endurance.

Start with *Nadisodhan Pranayama* and meditation within a day or two of delivery. After one week add *Pawan Muktasana* series and after another week you can resume your normal yogic routine, if the childbirth was normal.

Shahjoli should be added to tone up the slackened pelvic floor and *agnisara kriya* to tighten the abdominal muscles.

Shahjoli

Technique:
- Sit in *Padmasana* or *Ardha Padmasana*.
- Contract the pelvic muscles.
  (The act is similar to what you do to control urination)
- Hold the contraction for a few seconds.
- Release.
- Repeat 50 times.

You can synchronise the contraction with your breathing in the following manner.
- Contract with inhalation.
- Release with exhalation.

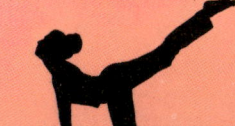

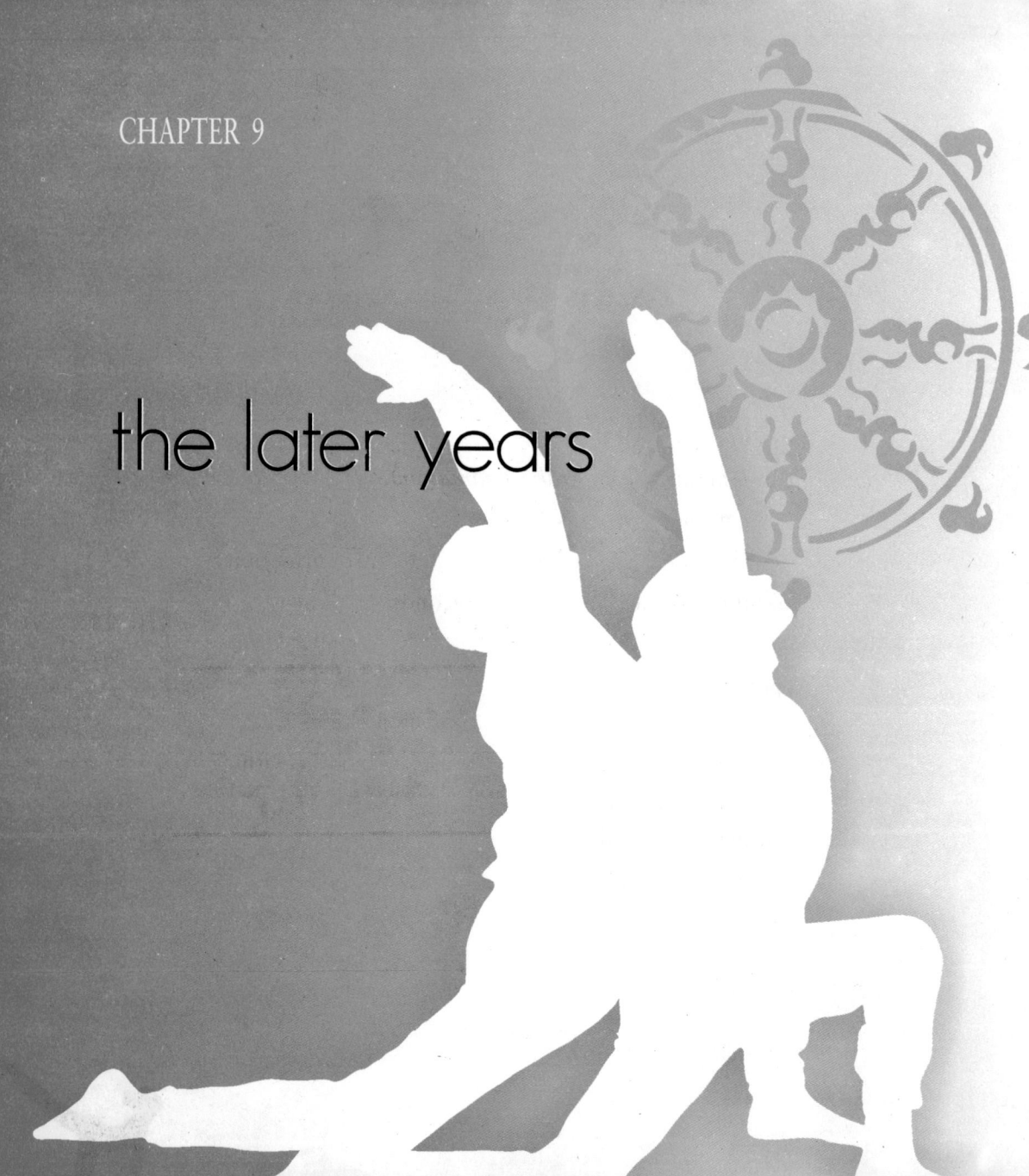

CHAPTER 9

the later years

THE LATER YEARS

The vedic man's lifespan was supposed to be a hundred years, out of which the second half was meant to be spent in near isolation. The first part of this phase was called *Vanaprastha ashrama* in which he gradually withdrew from active life. He retired to the forest with his spouse to lead a simple life, catering to his own needs. He spent his time in spiritual pursuit, studying scriptures and listening to saints and spiritual masters. He did not completely cut off ties with society and returned to his family from time to time. But the last phase known as *Sanyasa ashrama* required him to renounce the world completely. He dedicated himself wholeheartedly to attain his spiritual goal - salvation.

To live alone without drugs, doctors, nurses and attendants needs the highest degree of physical and mental strength which the vedic man must have possessed and which man today unfortunately lacks. Today, as the modern man crosses his fifty years, he is plagued by a number of degenerating maladies such as:

Failing eyesight: with advancing age the eyes lose their elasticity, especially of the lenses, making focusing on objects a short distance away difficult.

Glaucoma: another eye problem of

the elderly where fluid accumulates in the eyeballs. This puts pressure on the delicate optic tissues, causing pain. Untreated, this condition can lead to blindness.

Hearing loss: It is common to start losing hearing sensitivity from the twenties. The degeneration is very slow in the beginning, making it unnoticeable, but after sixty-five it can accelerate.

Skin Problems: The skin becomes dry, itchy and spotty. Weak oil-producing sebaceous glands, less blood supply to the skin, nutritional deficiencies and over-exposure to the sun's ultraviolet rays are responsible for these problems.

Enlarged Prostate: This is a common occurrence in older men. As the prostate gland surrounds the urethra (the duct through which urine passes) its swelling can interfere with free urination. One may get up several times during the night to pass urine. With such disturbed sleep, the body's degeneration is bound to accelerate.

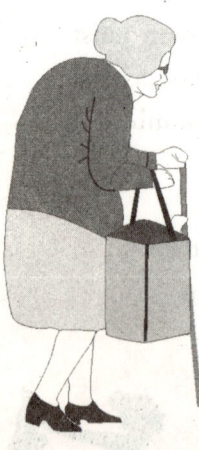

Osteoporosis: The meaning of osteoporosis is porous bones. The stored calcium in the bones decreases over time resulting in this disorder. The skeleton weakens and becomes prone to fractures. The bones can break with a little or no unusual strain.

Generally, one out of every four women above the age of forty-five, and nine out of ten women older than seventy-five suffer from this aliment. During the first five years after menopause, a woman may lose as much as twenty-five per cent of her bone mass. It is because the production of estrogen, the hormone which helps in the formation of healthy bones, drops during and after menopause. For men this problem is not so acute.

Memory loss: The brain cells start dying in the elderly at a fast rate. This results in memory loss or dementia. One's intellectual and social abilities can also be affected adversely causing many problems for the sufferer as well as the people around him.

Alzheimer's disease: The most serious of all old-age problems, due to which the brain cells die at a faster rate, is Alzheimer's disease. The sufferer loses his memory rapidly, leading to irritability, anxiety, depression, confusion and restlessness and then progressive disintegration of personality, judgement and social graces. Later, the person remembers nothing and recognises nobody.

Various factors, such as toxic exposure, viruses,

neurochemical abnormalities and genetic factors are thought to be the causes of this dreaded disease. High blood pressure and elevated cholesterol can also trigger off the ailment.

The ancient Indians followed a lifestyle prescribed by the vedas which may not be practical to practise in today's world, but by practising yoga - the ancient system of wellbeing - one can attempt to prevent all the above mentioned maladies.

Yoga slows down the body's degeneration considerably while improving tissue regeneration. Many yoga practitioners retain their memory, senses, agility of the body and mind in their old age. One should take up yoga from an early age for the best results.

After the thirties the practices meant for the young adult should be added to the yogic routine. People who have never practised yoga till their forties or fifties, should follow the author's book *Yoga for Busy People*. If they are older, they should consult a competent yoga teacher. *Pawanmuktasana* series of asanas contained in the above mentioned book can be practised at any age. Start with three rounds only, gradually increasing to ten rounds.

The following yogic techniques are meant to prevent problems related to aging.

For The Eyes

EXERCISE I

Technique:
- Lift your fists with the thumbs free and pointing up, to your shoulder level about three feet away from each other (you should be able to see the left thumb with your right eye and the right thumb with the left eye).

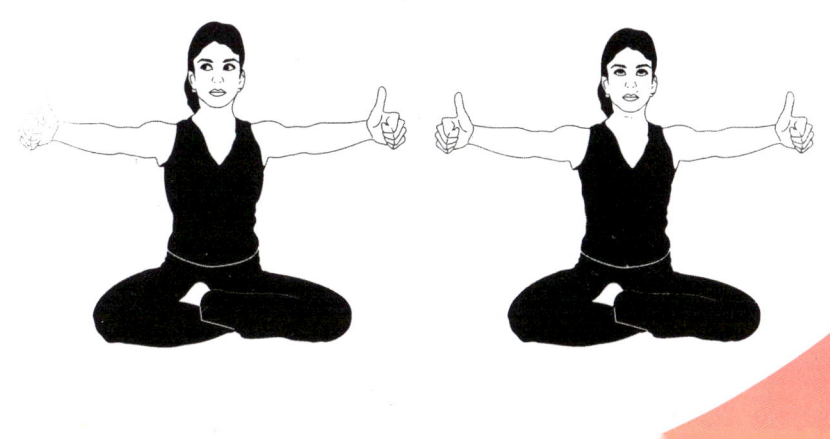

- Look at the left thumb for five counts.
- Look up at the centre of your eyebrows by crossing the eyes.
- Hold for five counts.
- Look at the right thumb for five counts and again look at the centre for five counts.
- Repeat ten times.
- Close eyes for half a minute.

EXERCISE II

Technique:
- Place the right hand as in the last exercise.
- Place the left hand down and straight in front.
- Look at the left thumb for five counts, then look at the right thumb for five counts.
- Repeat ten times.
- Change the hands and repeat ten times.
- Close eyes for half a minute.

EXERCISE III

Technique:
- Put out the right fist in front and move the arm in a circle following the thumb with your eyes.
- Repeat five times.
- Move the arm anti-clockwise while looking at the thumb.
- Repeat five times.
- Practise the same with your left arm.

EXERCISE IV

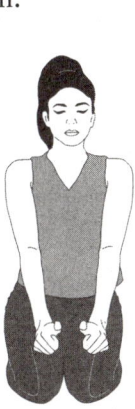
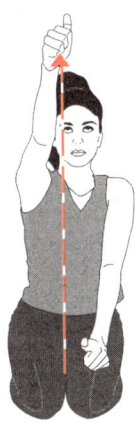

Technique:
- Hold your right hand in front and slowly move it up and down with your eyes fixed on the thumb.
- Repeat ten times.
- Practise with the left hand.

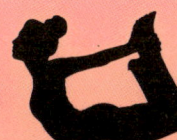

EXERCISE V

Technique:

This exercise should be practised outdoors, looking at a distant tree or better at a star at night.

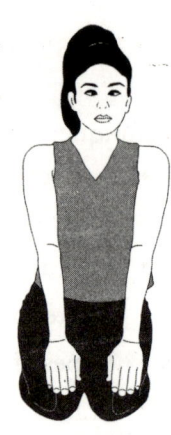

- Look at a distant object and the tip of your nose alternatively.
- Practise it 10-15 times.

After the above exercise and after the daily yogic practices, rub your hands together till they are warm, then place the palms lightly on your closed eyes. The enhanced energy flow due to *yogasanas* energises the optic muscles and nerves.

Important: *Neti* prevents many disorders of the eyes. It should be practised two to three times a week.

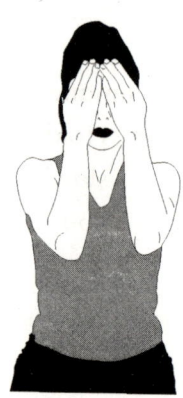

Vajroli

This practice prevents all prostate problems.

Technique:
- Sit in *Vajrasana*.
- Contract the muscles as you do to control urination.
- Hold for ten counts.
- Release the contraction.
- Repeat 50 times.

To prevent osteoporosis *Surya Namaskar* is most effective. *Parvatasan* which is the fifth step of *Suryanamaskar* and *Trikonasana* are also excellent.

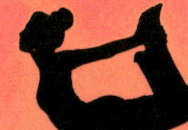

Trikonasana

Technique:

- Stand with your feet apart and arms out sideways at the shoulder level.
- Exhaling, bend to the right and touch the right foot with the right hand.
- Inhaling, return to the starting position.
- Repeat on the left side. Repeat ten times.

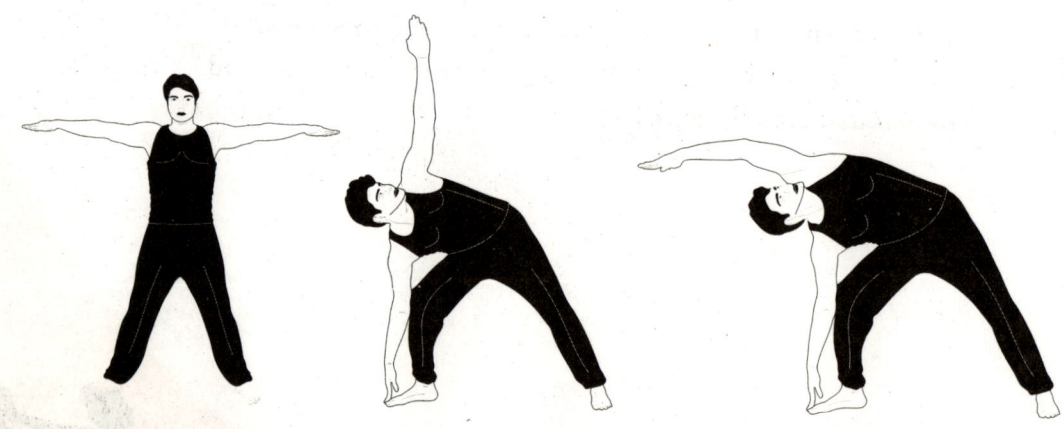

A diet rich in calcium is essential for strong bones. As Vitamin D is needed for proper use of this mineral, spending some time in the sun everyday is necessary. Also, too much meat and dairy products should be avoided. They turn the blood acidic reducing calcium from bones.

Bhramari Pranayama maintains the health of the ears keeping one's hearing sharp till the end, while all dynamic *asanas* are good for the skin.

For a sharp memory all inverted asanas such as *Sarvangasana* are excellent, as they bring a rich supply of blood to the brain.

Shashankasana can be substituted for people who cannot practise inverted *asanas*.

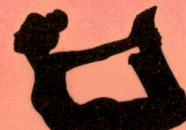

The following mental exercises are also recommended.
(i) Study and memorise a verse from a scripture.

धर्मक्षेत्रे कुरुक्षेत्रे समवेता युयुत्सवः ।
मामकाः पाण्डवाश्चैव किमकुर्वत सञ्जय ॥

Dhrtarastra said: O Sanjay what did my sons desirous of battle and the sons of Pandu do after assembling at the holy land of righteousness Kurukshetra?

(ii) Think of words or names starting with the same letter.
(iii) From a pack of playing cards take out four cards. Look at them carefully, turn them upside down and try to remember them. Check if you are correct. When you remember ten such sets without a mistake, increase the number of cards from four to five. Go on increasing the number as your memory improves.
(iv) Observe your surroundings for some time. Then close your eyes and remember them in detail.

(v) Mentally repeat "my memory is becoming stronger by the day", several times in a day.
(vi) Recollect a past event in detail.
(vii) Remember a few landmarks while going somewhere and check them out while returning.

CHAPTER 10

meditation and its nuances

MEDITATION AND ITS NUANCES

Stress is an integral part of life. Human beings have always experienced it – from birth to the end of their lives. Some may feel it more and some less but none can escape it. And stress harms the system as nothing else does. It has been seen that during times of stress 50,000 IU of Vitamin A is depleted from the body in ten minutes, which means, even the healthiest person can be deficient in this vitamin in under two hours of stress. In the long run, stress causes immense damage to the body, mind and psyche resulting in wide and varied ailments and disorders.

To release stress, many methods have been devised the world over. Meditation is one and probably the most accepted. There are innumerable types of meditation, all equally effective. One needs to choose the right meditation to derive its full benefits. Importantly, the meditation must suit the temperament and limitations of the person attempting it. It is wrong of teachers to emphasise on one kind of meditation for all. For instance, for a *rajasic* person who is basically restless, sitting still and concentrating on an object is almost impossible. In trying to do so, he may feel more restless and his mind may run amock. The more he tries to keep his body and mind still, the more rebellious they become and in the process more tension is created. Similarly, a *tamasic* person may find it difficult to remain awake when he closes his eyes for meditation. Only a *saatwik* person can practise any type of meditation including the classic method of sitting still and concentrating on an object or symbol. *Tratak* and *likhit japa* (written *mantra*) are more suitable for a *tamasic* person as these can be done with the eyes open while a *rajasic* person can succeed in a *tantric* meditation or mantra meditation.

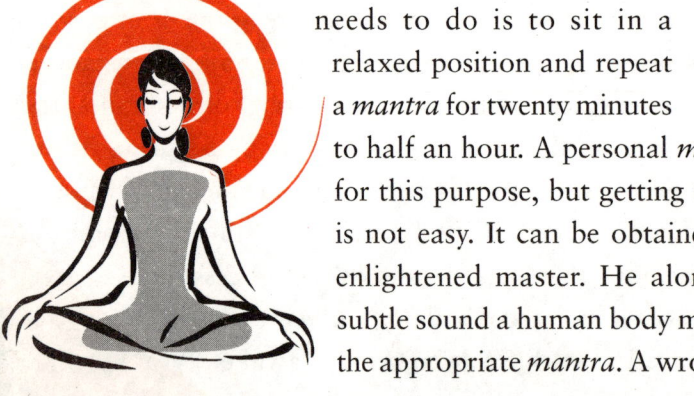

Mantra meditation suits all types of people and is easy to practise. In this meditation, it is not mandatory to sit in an upright meditative posture nor is it necessary to keep the eyes closed. All one needs to do is to sit in a relaxed position and repeat a *mantra* for twenty minutes to half an hour. A personal *mantra* is the best for this purpose, but getting the right *mantra* is not easy. It can be obtained only from an enlightened master. He alone can hear the subtle sound a human body makes and choose the appropriate *mantra*. A wrong one can clash with one's inner sound and create discord leading to irreversible damage to the body or mind. Once a personal *mantra* is practised, it should not be changed, as the sound vibration of the *mantra* permeates every cell in the system and a new *mantra* can only create chaos and confusion both in the mind and the body. In case a personal *mantra* is not available, a universal mantra such as *Soham,* and *Om* or a religious one such as *Om namah Shivaya, Om Manipadme Hum, Arhint, Vahe guru, Asham Vohu,* Hail Mary or Amen can be safely used. And they are all very effective.

Long hours of meditation should be avoided as it strains the heart, which has to supply extra blood to the brain for its extra activities during the practice. Secondly, lengthy meditation creates depression in the nervous system. One may become sensitive to sounds, introverted and withdrawn. Lastly, the body's inner temperature, so vital for proper digestion, falls during prolonged meditation, which may lead to ailments such as dyspepsia, rheumatism, arthritis and cancer.

Lack of oxygen in the system during long hours of meditation may lead to depression, while hyperacidity in the stomach gives rise to illusions and hallucinations.

Meditation should not be practised alone but in conjunction with *hatha* yoga for various reasons. First, as it increases the mental energy, it may lead to an imbalance in the energy system bringing about behavioural changes at times unacceptable to people around. Secondly *hatha* yoga rectifies certain conditions of the body which obstruct meditation. For example, if there are aches and pains in the body, the mind will be thinking of them rather than focusing on the object of concentration. Numbness in the legs is also a great hindrance. If they become numb during meditation, the practice will come to an end. Continuing the practice with numb legs can, in the long run, result in paralysis of the legs. However, moving the body during meditation is no meditation at all and will give none of its benefits. Hence, meditation should be balanced with the right *asanas*, *pranayama* and *shatkarma* in the right proportion. A practical combination is one hour of *hatha* yoga and half an hour of meditation.

Choose your meditation well after trying a few different methods, and practise it regularly at the same time every day. The body and mind like it that way.

SOME TECHNIQUES FOR CHILDREN

I. Music Meditation

Play some instrumental music and ask the child to listen to only one instrument for five minutes. One day you may ask him to follow the flute, another day the drum and yet another day the violin. After five minutes, play *sa re ga ma* (do re me sa) in an instrument and ask him to sing. Instead of *sa re ga*, he should say *Om-Om-Om*.

II. Colour Meditation

Ask the child to mentally visualise the alphabets in different colours. For example, 'a' in blue, 'b' in green etc. Let the child follow your suggestions with his eyes closed.

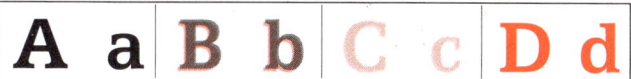

After 4 to 5 minutes, he should open his eyes and visualise his surroundings in one colour. For example, he should imagine the trees in pink, sky in pink etc. Use only pastel colours.

Alternatively, show him coloured objects, one at a time and ask him to close his eyes and imagine them. Use objects from nature – a leaf, flower, coloured stones, fruits etc.

III. Matter

Ask the child to imagine a material in all shapes and sizes. For example if you choose earth, then let the child imagine it in various forms – pitcher, glass, lamp, mud hut and the likes.

Other materials can be water, gold, silver, cotton, wool, precious stones etc.

(You should not use the colour black, violent sea, storm and moon in any of the above techniques; choose mild and soothing things).

IV. Mantra Meditation

A *guru* can choose a *mantra*, or teach the child the *Gayatri Mantra* which he should repeat for five to ten minutes.

SOME TECHNIQUES FOR ADOLESCENTS

Sit in a comfortable position and make no movement.

Close your eyes. Move your mind over the body and search for sensations – itching, irritation, throbbing, pain etc. Move from sensation to sensation dwelling only a few seconds on each one but with a kind of non-involvement. After two to three minutes, feel your breath in the nostrils. Mentally repeat 'peace' while inhaling and 'strength' while exhaling. (you can use other words if you like). Practise it for four to five minutes.

Be aware of all that passes before your closed eyes – colours, figures, forms and objects. After two to three minutes, take a deep breath and chant *Ommm* or just mmmm as you exhale and concentrate on the sound. Repeat three times, be aware of your surroundings and open your eyes.

Rub your hands well and place the palms lightly on your eyes for ten seconds or so. Repeat three times and open your eyes.

SOME TECHNIQUES FOR ADULTS

Tratak

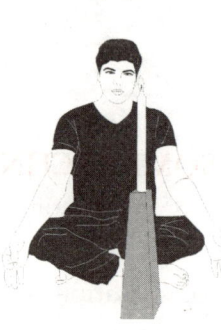

Technique:

Keep a lighted candle in front of you at an arm's distance and at your eye level. Sitting still in the meditative position, stare at the flame for three minutes or till your eyes water. Close eyes and concentrate on the image of the flame in your mind till it fades (around two minutes). Open your eyes. Repeat it twice more.

Chakra visualisation

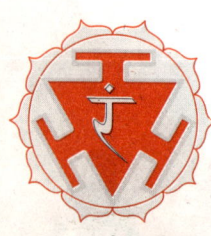

Sit still and straight in a meditative pose such as *padmasana* or *sukhasana* (cross-legged) and concentrate on your natural breaths. Say to yourself mentally 'I am breathing in, I am breathing out' for two to three minutes. Now, imagine you are breathing from the left nostril, breathing out from the right; then breathing in from the right and breathing out from the left. Continue for another five to six minutes. Then imagine you are breathing from the navel. When you inhale, imagine the breath entering the navel to go to the *manipura chakra* on the spine behind that spot, then comes out of the navel as you exhale. After the rhythm is well established, repeat the *mantra Ram* (र्) mentally. *Ram* as you inhale and again *Ram* as you exhale. Breathe slowly and deeply. You can hold the breath for a second after inhalation and visualise the *manipura chakra*. Repeat the above process with the following *chakras* spending 2 to 3 minutes on each one.

    Anahata - behind the heart   Mantra - yam
    Visuddhi - behind the throat   Mantra – ham
    Ajna - behind the center of the eyebrows   Mantra – om

Finally, concentrate on a symbol, keeping it either in your heart or in between the eyebrows. The symbol may come spontaneously to your mind or may be a chosen one. Choose your symbol from a deity, your *guru*, a saint, a flower, a star, a tiny flame, the cross, *trishul*, *shivalinga* or any other object which can hold your attention and can invoke divine feelings in you. If the mind wanders, follow it for a while and then gently bring it back to the object. Practise it for five minutes or so and then take your mind out to the surroundings, be aware of your body, and slowly open your eyes.

FOR THE ELDERLY (optional)

Nama Smaran

Choose a name of God or a deity and mentally repeat it with each breath. While inhaling say it once and while exhaling also do the same. You may or may not sit in a meditative pose but try to keep the body still.

Reflecting on nature is also a good form of meditation for the old. For this you have to be in the open, sitting relaxed and in a comfortable position. Be aware of each thing around you and reflect on it for some time before moving on to another one. For example, notice a tree – see how the leaves are dancing, observe the flowers, try to get the smell, imagine the touch – soft and velvety. Feel the presence of divinity in it. Let your heart open up to it. Feel joy and love flooding your heart. Then move on to something else and do the same.

FOR PREGNANT WOMEN
(the first five months)

- Sit in *Padmasana* (lotus pose) or *Sukhasana*.
- Chant *Om* 27 times.

- Concentrate on the rise and fall of the navel for about 10 minutes. Visualise a golden womb either inside your abdomen or outside the body. Visualise a sleeping baby and its various parts in detail. Imagine that you touch the baby and it wakes up, looks at you and smiles. Visualise it turning to a sound. Imagine yourself putting a little honey in its mouth which the baby licks happily. Then it plays for some time kicking its arms and legs and after a while goes back to sleep.
- If you want to inculcate a particular virtue in your child you can do so from the fourth month. Suppose you want your child to be brave, mentally repeat 'bravery' for two to three minutes. Then remember some brave people you know or have read about and wish to have the child as brave.
- Now visualise a sun behind your navel and concentrate on it for two to three minutes.
- Chant *Om* seven times and open your eyes.

In the latter half of the pregnancy, it may become difficult to sit in a meditative pose. One should then sit in a relaxed position and practise mantra meditation.

CHAPTER 11

yoganidra

YOGANIDRA

Yoganidra is a beautiful experience. Every time it is conducted, the practitioners express their wonder and satisfaction. *Yoganidra* takes one to the most relaxed state where one is neither completely asleep nor fully awake. One just drifts in and out of a semiconscious state. For some though, it is almost impossible to remain awake. I remember my friend Indira, who would go off to sleep within a few minutes and would wake up when the session was over. I wanted her to experience it properly, and told her to try harder to stay awake, but she just could not. I suggested she sat on a sofa to do *Yoganidra*. That didn't help either; she kept dosing throughout the practice. Finally, I made her sit on a settee with no back-rest. She still slept!

Yoganidra has the same effect on children too. Janet, an English lady, had once brought her seven-year-old daughter to me. She was very worried as the child was not sleeping well. She would not fall asleep easily and when she did she would toss and turn all through the night. I made her do *Yoganidra*. No sooner had I started saying it, she became still, and very soon was fast asleep. Even after I stopped saying, she would not wake up. Much later, Janet had to shake the little

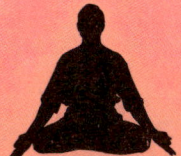

girl to awaken her! She was amazed and could not believe her eyes!

Every day young or old, every body should practise *Yoganidra*. Ten minutes of *Yoganidra* at the end of the day removes all tension from the body and mind and induces sound sleep. Though a live voice is the most effective for this purpose, a recorded one can be used for convenience. *Yoganidra* text should be spoken slowly and softly giving pauses at the right places. It should be recited like a poem rather than spoken plainly.

Technique

SOME OPTIONS FOR CHILDREN

OPTION 1

'Close your eyes – imagine you are standing before a mirror. In the mirror you first look at your right hand, - right arm, - right waist, - right hip, - right thigh, - right knee, right foot, left hand, left arm, left waist, left hip, left thigh, left knee, left foot, top of the head, forehead, eyes, nose, lips, chin, neck, chest, stomach. Everything is just perfect.

Now imagine it is early evening – you are walking in a park – see a tree full of yellow flowers – you spot a swing – sit on it and start swinging. You are swinging higher and higher – It feels so nice. From the swing you spot a small pond. You stop swinging, get off and walk towards the pond. You sit on a rock near the pond and keep looking at the clear blue water. You throw a pebble and see the tiny waves. Now it is becoming slightly dark. You see a fairy coming towards you holding a candle in her hand. She is smiling and is coming closer and closer. Now she is standing right in front. You see her beautiful radiant face. She now says 'My child I will grant you a wish. You just close your eyes and say it three times'. So you close your eyes and say your wish three times in your mind.
Then, you find yourself in your house in your own room. And whatever you had wished for has come true ——— (pause)

Move your hands a little – move your arms - your feet – legs stretch and open your eyes'.

OPTION 2

'Close your eyes and relax. Imagine you are in a field to play your favourite game. Your favourite player has come to teach you how to play well.

He first gives you a cream to apply on every part of your body saying it is an energizing cream. So you apply it to your right hand, right arm, right side of the body, right thigh, right knee, right foot, left hand, left arm, left side, left hip, left thigh, left knee, left foot, forehead, cheeks, chin, neck, chest and abdomen.

Your coach now asks you to lie down on your back for a while. You lie down and look at the sky. You see many coloured kites. You watch them ——(pause). You hear somebody whispering – 'If you spot a violet kite, make a wish and repeat it three times in your mind. It will come true. And lo – you see a violet kite. So you quickly close your eyes and mentally repeat your wish. Your coach tells you that you should go home and come back the next day after the cream has made the body strong. You are already feeling stronger. You go home and realise that your wish has come true. You are so happy. Move your feet, hands, legs, head, stretch and open your eyes.'

SOME OPTIONS FOR ADULTS

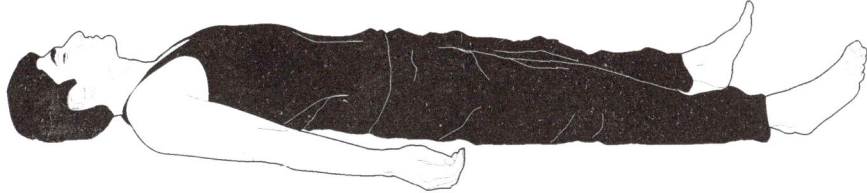

Lie down in *Shavasana* (as above). Close your eyes gently. Say to yourself mentally 'I am going to relax completely. – I will experience deep relaxation. – I am going to practise yoganidra which will give me the best possible relaxation.' Now say 'relax' and relax the body. Go on repeating 're – la – x, re – la – x" and feel your body relaxing more and more. Make a resolution and repeat it three times in your mind. Now take your mind to all the body parts to feel the deep relaxation while mentally saying the name of that part in the following sequence.

Right thumb, index finger, middle finger, ring finger, little finger, palm, wrist, elbow, shoulder, right armpit, right hip, thigh, knee, calf, ankle, foot, the big toe, second toe, third toe, fourth toe, fifth toe.

Repeat the same with the left side.

Right shoulder, left shoulder, back, back of the head, top of the head, forehead, right eyebrow, left eyebrow, right eye, left eye, upper lip, lower lip, chin, neck, chest, stomach, abdomen.

Right leg, left leg, right arm, left arm, the whole of the front, the whole of the back, the whole body – the whole body.

Imagine it is the height of summer – it is extremely hot – you are in a hot room – you are feeling very hot – you are perspiring profusely ———

Now imagine your are in a hill station – it is winter – you are feeling very cold – and watching the snowfall. All around is white – more white.

Now visualize – a flowing river and a boat, a sea with big waves – stars at night – full moon – a pink lotus – blue sky – candle flame.

Repeat your resolution three times in your mind, be aware of the external sounds, be aware of your body, move it slowly, stretch and slowly open your eyes.

ADDITIONAL PRACTICE FOR THE OLD
(optional)

Before ending the session – say mentally 'I am forgiving all the people who have hurt me and insulted me. They are ignorant people. Let God show them the right path. I have forgiven them, which has made me receptive to the divine energy. Now I feel God's energy and blessings flowing through me.'

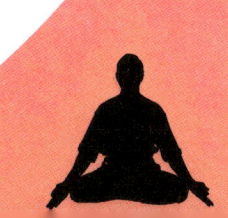

CHAPTER 12

nourishment

NOURISHMENT

Highly evolved yogis may not need food to be alive as they can absorb all they need from the atmosphere. But for ordinary mortals, how healthy a person is depends primarily on what he or she eats. Yoga and other health systems can work better when the food requirements of the body are met. Body tissues need continual replacement of nutrients; different body parts needing different nutrients to be healthy. Also the nutrients depend on one another to carry out their function properly. They are not effective in the absence of specific other nutrients. For example, iron can be absorbed only in the presence of Vitamin C. And as this vitamin cannot be stored in the body, unless it is taken regularly, one might get iron deficient ailments inspite of taking food rich in this mineral. Hence all the categories of food must be included in one's diet. Food deficiency can lead to wide and varied problems including some peculiar ones, as can be seen from the following.

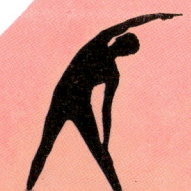

Symptoms	Deficiency
Excessive thirst	Sodium
Cramps	Sodium, Calcium, Iron, Vitamin B Pantothenic Acid
Breathlessness	Sodium, Iron, Pantothenic Acid
Drowsiness	Sodium
Confusion	Sodium
Obesity	Calcium, Iron
Paleness	Calcium
Listless	Calcium, Iron, B1, B2, Biotin
Sensitivity to cold	Calcium, Iron
Hallucination	Calcium, B12
Fear	Calcium
Poor concentration	Calcium
Anaemia	Calcium, iron, Folic Acid, Tryptophan
Lower back-ache	Calcium, Iron
Acidity	Calcium
Kidney & liver problem	Calcium

Insomnia	Iron, B1
Sore mouth	Iron, B2, B12, Niacin
Heavy head	Iron
Pimples	Vitamin A
Scaly skin	Vitamin A
Ageing	Vitamin A
Loss of appetite	Vitamins B1, B2, B6, B12, Folic Acid
Loss of interest	Vitamin B1
Suicidal	Vitamins B1, B12
Constipation	Vitamin B1
Gastritis	Inositol
Pins and needles	B1, B12, Iron, Biotin
Muscle weakness	Biotin
Retarded growth	Pantothenic Acid, Folic Acid
Loss of weight	Pantothenic Acid
Rheumatoid Arthritis	Pantothenic Acid
Burning in throat and stomach after food	Niacin
Sick feeling after non-vegetarian food	Niacin

Weak mind	Folic Acid
Joint pain	Vitamin C
Desire for sour food	Vitamin B12
Loss of hair	Tin, Iron and Vitamin B
Depression	Vitamins B1, B12, Tryptophan
Sensitivity to light	Vitamin B2
Stress	Vitamin B2, Tryptophan
Diarrhoea	Folic Acid

It has been seen that the body does not utilise synthetic vitamins well. Also the high concentration may even harm the system. Therefore, vitamins and minerals should be taken in the natural form. Care should be taken to replenish nutrients before they are used up, as our system can store them for limited periods only. It can store Vitamin A and D for six months; K only a few days; E somewhere in between; B and C, hardly at all and protein not at all.

DAILY REQUIREMENTS

Nutrients	Adult
Carbohydrates	around 400 g
Protein	Sedentary – around 50 g
	Pregnancy & lactation- 100 g
Fat	6 tsp
Iron	10-15 mg
Calcium	500-600 mg
Sodium	10 g
Iodine	150 mcg
Copper	2 mg
	3 mg (pregnancy)
Magnesium	5 mg per kg body weight
Manganese	5 mg
Zinc	6-15 mg
Vitamin A	2500 – 7500 IU
Vitamin D	500 IU
Vitamin E	15 mg
Vitamin B1	0.5 – 1.5 mg
Vitamin B2	around 2 mg

Vitamin B6	2- 4 mg
Vitamin B12	0.5 – 2.8 mcg
Folic Acid	50 – 100 mcg
Vitamin C	70 – 75 mg
Vitamin K	1 –2 mg
Nicotinic Acid	around 20 mg
Pantothenic Acid	10 –15 mg

RICH SOURCES

Food	Quantity	Value
Proteins		
Milk	½ kg	18 g
Egg	1	7 g
Soyabean	½ cup	38 g
Peas	½ cup	29 g
Chicken	200 g	23 g
Calcium		
Milk	1 cup	300 mg
Sardine	50 g	200 mg

Methi Leaves	50 g	210 mg
Cheese	50 g	350 mg
Crab	50 g	600 mg
Mint	50 mg	220 mg

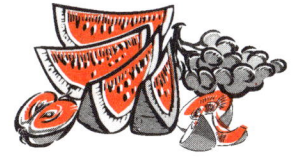

Phosphorus

Milk	30% of weight
Chicken	30% of weight
Cereal	13% of weight
Vegetables	10% of weight
Beans	5% of weight
Egg	5% of weight
Fruits	4% of weight

Iron

Liver	50 g	5 mg
Yolk	50 g	6 mg
Ragi	50 g	8 mg
Coriander Leaves	50 g	9 mg
Chaulai	50 g	13 mg
Spinach	50 g	20 mg

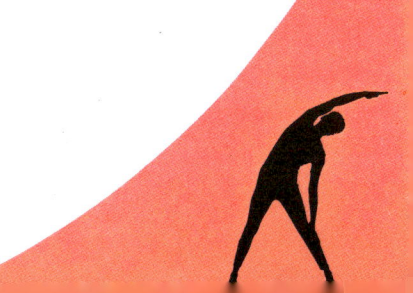

Potassium

Figs	50 g	500 mg
Almonds	50 g	400 mg
Walnut	50 g	350 mg
Liver	50 g	200 mg
Fish	50 g	150 mg
Chicken	50 g	200 mg
Banana	50 g	175 mg
Peas	50 g	150 mg
Grapes	50 g	125 mg

Vitamin A

Cord Liver oil	50 g	100000 IU
Carrot	50 g	10000 IU
Spinach	50 g	6500 IU
Liver	50 g	2000 IU
Butter	50 g	1750 IU
Cheese	50 g	750 IU
Lettuce	50 g	1000 IU
Sweet Potato	50 g	3000 IU

Vitamin D

Sufficient Vitamin D is produced in the body in the presence of sunlight. Certain foods such as fish, egg, liver, butter and milk are also rich source of Vitamin D.

Vitamin E

Wheatgerm	100 g	260 mg
Seasame seeds	100 g	30 mg
Palm	100 g	60 mg
Almond	100 g	40 mg
Soyabean	100 g	140 mg
Crab	100 g	50 mg

Vitamin B1

Peas	50 gm	180 mcg
Wheat	50 gm	180 mcg
Rice bran	50 gm	1350 mcg
Ragi	50 gm	100 mcg

Vitamin B2
Soyabean	50 mg	370 mcg
Gram	50 mg	200 mcg
Rice bran	50 mg	250 mcg

Vitamin B6
Wheat	50 mg	5 mcg
Pulses	50 mg	6 mcg
Yeast	50 mg	25 mcg

Vitamin B12
Liver	50 mg	50 mcg
Egg	50 mg	3 mcg
Fish	50 mg	5 mcg
Milk	½ ltr	2.4 mcg

Folic Acid
Spinach	50 g	40 mcg
Asparagus	50 g	25 mcg
Broccoli	50 g	12 mcg

Wheat	50 g	25 mcg
Peas	50 g	30 mcg

Nicotinic Acid

Whole wheat	50 g	3 mg
Liver	50 g	5 mg
Peanut	50 g	6 mg
Yeast	50 g	5 mg

Pantothenic Acid - Liver, chicken, egg, milk, soyabean, fish, tomato, peanut.

Vitamin C

Amla	50 g	500 mg
Orange	50 g	30 mg

Vitamin K - Green vegetables

All values are approximate only.

VEGETARIANISM AND NON-VEGETARIANISM

Though yoga prefers a vegetarian diet, *tantra*, whose offshoot is yoga, makes it mandatory to consume meat and fish. Ayurveda too speaks of the benefits of meat and fish. According to Indian scriptures even gods and *rishis* took meat. It is also said that as life started in the sea, everything of the sea is conducive to life and hence seafood, especially fish, must be taken for good health. Positive and negative points exist in everything so also in vegetarian and non-vegetarian food. What one eats should be one's personal choice.

Helpful Hints

1. Ginger juice should be added to cauliflower to avoid flatulence
2. Cabbage should be cooked with a little *heeng* (asafoetida) for the same purpose.
3. A piece of ginger should be chewed with a pinch of salt before meals to activate the digestive system.
4. 1 tsp pure malt vinegar mixed with a glass of water should be taken after eating meat to prevent most of the ill effects of meat consumption.

5. Yam should be cooked with tamarind leaves to inactivate its paralysis causing neurotoxins.
6. Fatty fish causes high acidity.
7. Prawns are digested easily if eaten with papaya.
8. Watermelon may cause indigestion when eaten with rice.
9. Cooking tomatoes and starchy food together is bad for the stomach.
10. Ripe jackfruit is digested easily if taken with honey and coconut.
11. Honey should be added to fruit if the latter causes distension.
12. A piece of mango peel should be eaten after taking mangoes to prevent indigestion
13. Fats should not be taken without carbohydrate as that can cause vomiting.

Conducive to life

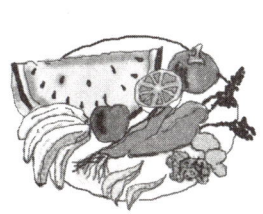
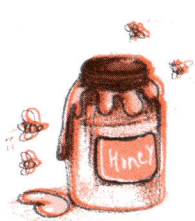

Honey with fruits prevents distension

CHAPTER 13

health facts

HEALTH FACTS

Acid-Alkaline balance: As long as this balance remains correct, most serious ailments are likely to stay away. It has been observed that cancer cells die in three hours if kept in an alkaline medium. Excess acid irritates the system and causes many diseases. Nutrients are not easily used in an acidic body. Acids increase in the body due to stress, rich diet, over-eating and excessive protein and sugar intake. Body produces alkaline substances which may not be adequate to neutralize all the acids. One can rectify that by taking plenty lot of alkaline food and by flushing out acids by drinking plenty lot of fluid.

Fasting: One of the functions of the liver is to detoxify the system. But at times, the toxins in the body are much in excess of the liver's capacity to eliminate them. This strains the liver gradually weakening it and leading to more toxins in the body. Fasting is an effective means to remove toxins. It also gives rest to the liver and rejuvenates it.

Clean Skin: The skin is a major toxin-removing organ. Through perspiration the skin throws out twelve ounces of impurity every day. When the water of the perspiration evaporates, the solid waste is left behind on the skin.

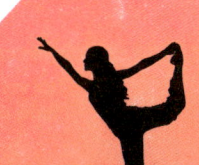

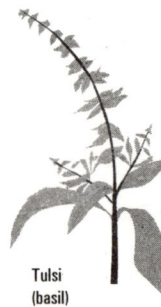

Tulsi (basil)

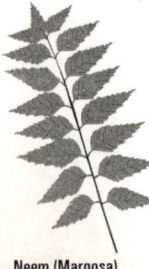

Neem (Margosa)

Tulsi and Neem Purify the air

It forms a thin coating and clogs the pores, preventing proper perspiration. Warm water bath with a good scrub is an effective way to keep the pores open.

Breathing right: Body tissues take up oxygen and nutrients from the blood and give off their waste products chiefly carbonic acid and urea which are injurious to the tissue health. Urea and other nitrogenous waste matter are removed by the kidneys, while carbonic acid is removed from the blood by the lungs, and is thrown out during exhalation. If the breathing is shallow, neither enough oxygen gets into the system nor is the carbonic acid effectively eliminated from it. Taking a few deep breaths every now and then is a wise move to rectify that.

Clean environment: Plants such as *tulsi* (basil) and *neem* (Margosa) near the house keep the air around you clean and fresh.

Happiness: A sad unhappy person may find it difficult to be healthy. So 'Be Happy!' Easier said than done. But you can at least repeat 'I am happy' which is easy said and easy done. It works!

SOME HEALTHY HABITS

Certain traditional practices promote good health. Try to include as many of them as possible.

1. Rise as early in the morning as you can, preferably before sun rise. After sunrise the body starts secreting acid. The later you get up the more acidic the system can become.
2. On rising, drink two glasses of water kept overnight in a copper vessel – People with a tendency to have gas may drink hot water instead.
3. Walk barefoot on grass for at least half an hour. It is supposed to strengthen the eyesight. Also it is said that the earth removes negative energy from the body through the soles.
4. Spend half an hour in the sun both morning and evening.
5. Massage mustard oil on each sole for 2-3 minutes in the morning. It strengthens the nervous system. If repeated at bed-time it induces sound sleep.
6. Massage *til* (Sesame seed) oil on the body before bath. It speeds up the blood circulation, removes gas and promotes lymphatic drainage from the system.

7. Face east while studying, eating or practising Yoga. You will absorb positive energy from the Sun.
8. While sleeping, the head should be towards the east so as not to clash with the Universal energy flow.

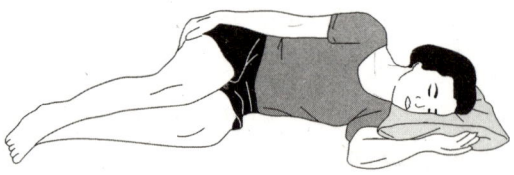

9. Sleeping on the left side facilitates better digestion.
10. Once a week take ½ tsp of raw turmeric powder in the morning in empty stomach. It destroys various harmful parasites and purifies the blood.
11. Eat a bitter tasting vegetable such as *karela* (bitter gourd) or *neem* (Margosa) leaves at lunch time for the same reason. Bitter food should not be taken at night.
12. One should not talk while eating as food can get into the wind pipe which many a time has proved fatal.
13. Drink water an hour before and after taking a meal.

PREVENTIVES

Cancer: 1 or 2 gm of turmeric powder in empty stomach. Also take an *amla* (Indian gooseberry) and a clove of garlic every day.

Conjunctivitis: Rub 3-4 crushed garlic cloves on your palms and place hands over your eyes for 2 minutes. Let the fume get into the eyes. Do it twice a day during an epidemic.

Deafness: Put a drop of mustard oil in each ear 2-3 times a week.

Diabetes: Drink ½ cup of bittergourd juice in the morning in empty stomach for one month every year.

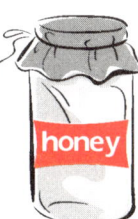

Enamel loss: Chew lettuce leaves after meals.

Heart ailments: amla, yeast and honey.

Infection of lungs, skin, kidneys and intestine: a clove of raw garlic daily.

Kidney ailments: turnip

Kidney stones: papaya, grapes and *kulthi*

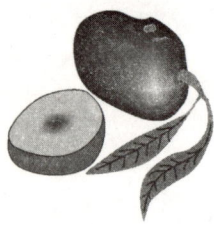

Malaria: 2 basil leaves and 2 pepper corns ground and taken on an empty stomach prevents this infection.
Osteoporosis: *Chaulai*, soya products, *til*, almond, dates.
Sunstroke: Mango
Tuberculosis (TB) - *Lauki*

Important: Yoga is a practical science and hence should be learnt under the direct supervision of an expert.

And remember: all rules work only if God wills it.

REFERENCES

1. Kristine M. Napier, *Eat to Heal*, Warner Books. 1998
2. Ann Wigmore, *Be Your Own Doctor*, Avery Publisher Group. 2nd Edition 1983.
3. Dr. Michael Sharon, *Nutrients A to Z*, Prion Books. 2004
4. Dr. Aman, *Medicinal Secrets of Your Food*.
5. J. D. Ritcliff, *I am Joe's Body*, Berkley Publishing Group, New York. 1982.
6. David E. Larson, *Mayo Clinic Family Health Book*, William Morrow & Company, Inc., New York. 1990.
7. Ernest R. Hilgard, Rita L. Atkinson and Richard C. Atkinson, *Introduction to Psychology*, Harcourt Brace Jovanorich Inc. 1979.
8. Robert A. Baron, *Psychology*, Prentice Hall College Division, 4th Edition. 1999.
9. Jose Silva and Philip Miele, *The Silva Mind Control Method*, Pocket Books. 1991.
10. Jose Silva with Robert B. Stone, *The Silva Mind Control Method For Getting Help From Your Other Side*, Pocket Books. 1989.

11. Swami Sivananda, *Health and Hygiene*, Divine Life Society. 6th Edition 1996.
12. Swami Sivananda, *Japa Yoga*, Divine Life Society. 11th Edition 1994.
13. Swami Sivananda, *Mind – Its Mysteries and Control*, Divine Life Society. 12th Edition 1994.
14. Swami Sivananda, *Sure Ways for Success in Life & God Realization*, Divine Life Society. 13th Edition 1990.
15. Swami Sivananda, *Concentration and Meditation*, Divine Life Society. 8th Edition 1990.
16. Yogi Ramacharaka, *Hatha Yoga*, Kessinger Publishing. 1998.
17. Yogi Ramacharaka, *Fourteen Lessons in Yogi Philosophy and Oriental Occultism*, Kessinger Publishing. 2003.
18. Paramahamsa Yogananda, *Autobiography of a Yogi*, Self Realisation Fellowship Publisher. 1979.
19. *Hatha Yoga Pradipika*, Bihar School of Yoga, Munger. 1985.
20. Swami Satyananda Saraswati, *Asana Pranayama Mudra Bandha*, Bihar School of Yoga, Munger. 2nd Edition 1971.

21. Swami Satyananda Saraswati, *Yoga Nidra,* Bihar School of Yoga, Munger.
22. Swami Satyananda Saraswati, *Meditation from Tantra*, Bihar School of Yoga, Munger. 5th Edition 1983.
23. Swami Satyananda Saraswati, *Self Realisation*, Bihar School of Yoga, Munger.
24. Swami Satyananda Saraswati, *Yogic Cure for Common Diseases*, Bihar School of Yoga, Munger. 1983.
25. *Teaching of Swami Satyananda Saraswati,* Bihar School of Yoga. Vol. I First Australian Edition 1981, Vol. IV 4th Enlarged Edition 1986 & Vol. V 1986.
26. Visnu Devananda, *Meditation and Mantras.*
27. Choa Kok Sui, *The Ancient Science & Art of Pranic Healing*, Institute for Inner Studies. 1987.
28. Swami Muktananda Saraswati, *Nawayogini Tantra.* 1975.
29. Swami Satyananda Saraswati, *Yoga Education for Children.* 1985.

INDEX

Ananda Madirasana	24	Padadhirasana	25
Ardhamatsyendrasana	58	Padahastasana	41
Bhadrasana	70	Padmasana (Lotus pose)	18
Bhramari Pranayama	19	Paschimottanasana	57
Chakki Chalana	68	Sarvangasana	54
Dhanurasana	50	Shahjoli	81
Dwikonasana	42	Shashanka Bhujangasana	44
Ekapada Pranamasana	26	Shashankasana	59
Gayatri Mantra	35	Shavasana	113
Kandhrasana	72	Simhasana	16
Lolasana	43	Surya Namaskar	32
Makarasana	17	Tadasana	40
Marjariasana	50	Tratak	104
Matsyasana	56	Trikonasana	92
Nadisodhana Pranayama	45	Titli	67
Namaskara	73	Utthanasana	70
Natavara	27	Vajroli	91
Nauka Sanchalana	69		

YOGA FOR BUSY PEOPLE
Bijoylaxmi Hota

Yoga for Busy People is a user-friendly book containing information necessary for maintaining good health, especially of a busy person who is likely to lose it the most. Good health is the outcome of exercise, rest and relaxation in the correct proportion, inner cleanliness, intake of essential nutients, avoidance of harmful substances and a stress-free mind. It is best achieved through asana (yogic exercise), pranayama (yogic breathing), shatkarma (cleansing techniques), yoganidra (yogic sleep) and meditation.

Apart from recommending the simplest yogic techniques that can be practised with ease by anyone, the book also shows how to fit them all into one's busy schedule.

YOGA TO BANISH BACKACHE
Bijoylaxmi Hota

Yoga To Banish Backache familiarises the reader with causes of various types of back pain such as cervical spondilitis, slipped disc, sciatica prolapse, intestinal gas and scoliosis and recommends simple yet effective yogic and natural remedies.

The author Bijoylaxmi Hota, is a yoga therapist of repute with more than twenty-five years of experience. She has successfully treated various ailments ranging from asthma, arthritis, and high blood pressure to tumour and cancer.

Bijoylaxmi Hota conducts yoga workshops within and outside India, has penned articles and produced TV programmes on the subject and has scripted dance recitals based on Indian philosophy.

YOGA FOR EVERYBODY
Bharti Joshi

Among the many kinds of yoga described by the philosopher sage Patanjali, *hatha yoga* is the practice of physical postures. The word *hatha* denotes the complementary nature of all things in the cosmos. *Yoga for Everybody* deals with this classic form of yoga whose practice helps achieve physical, mental, emotional and spiritual harmony, along with meditation, mantra repetition and breathing exercises. It starts with the importance of prayer in yoga and moves on to beginning exercises and then illustrates in detail the complete routine. It also dwells on *Suryanamaskar*, classification of *yogasans* (separating meditation postures from relaxation and action postures), *yoga trataka* and yogic breathing, ending with a chapter on *pranayama*. *Yoga for Everybody* is thus an exhaustive, one-stop guide to health through *hatha yoga*.

Bharati Joshi is a yoga enthusiast and practitioner of *hatha yoga* for the last 25 years. She has received her training and certification from Yoga Vidyadham, Pune and has also passed the Yoga Teachers Training course from Kaivalyadham, Lonavala. She has conducted yoga classes, especially for women, in Pune, Kolhapur and even abroad.

YOGA TO PRESERVE YOUTH AND BEAUTY
Bijoylaxmi Hota

Yoga to Preserve Youth and Beauty contains yogic, Vedic, Ayurvedic and traditional methods to develop a well-toned, well-proportional trim body, flawless glowing skin, shiny bright eyes, healthy bouncy hair and most importantly, inner composure – factors essential to remain beautiful, youthful and peaceful for life.

The author, Bijoylaxmi Hota, is a yoga therapist of repute with almost two and a half decades of experience. She has successfully treated various ailments ranging from asthma, arthritis, backache to tumours and cancer.